THE REMINISCENCE SKILLS TRAINING HANDBOOK

THE

REMINISCENCE SKILLS TRAINING HANDBOOK

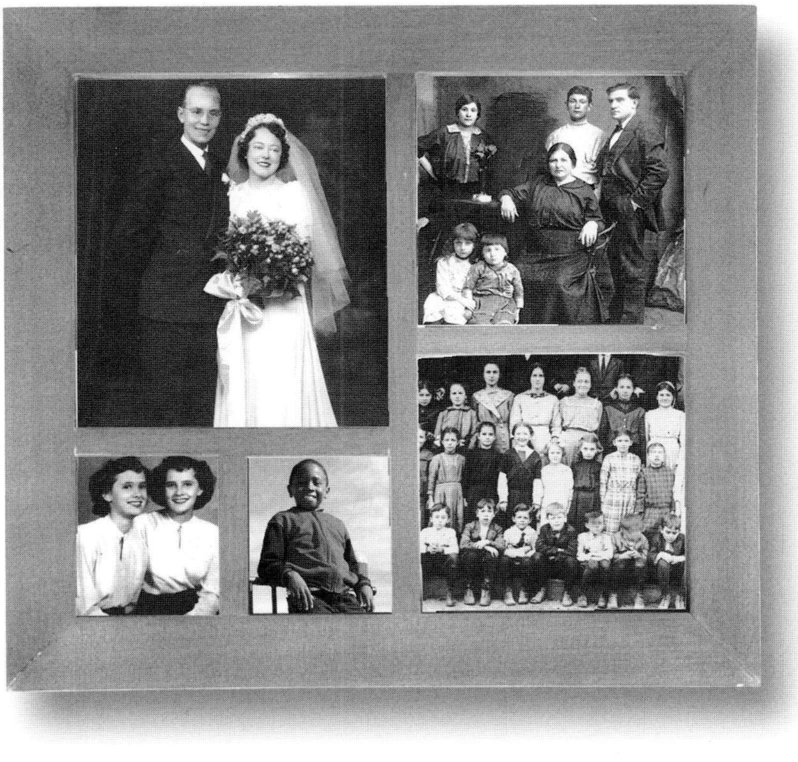

Ann Rainbow

Speechmark

www.speechmark.net

First published in 2003 by
Speechmark Publishing Ltd, 70 Alston Drive, Bradwell Abbey, Milton Keynes MK13 9HG, UK
Tel: +44 (0) 1908 326944 Fax: +44 (0) 1908 326960
www.speechmark.net

Reprinted 2008

002-5025/Printed in the United Kingdom/1030

British Library Cataloguing in Publication Data
Rainbow, Ann
The Reminiscence Skills Training Handbook
1. Reminiscing in old age – Therapeutic use 2. Reminiscing – Therapeutic use
I. Title
615.8'51'0846

ISBN 978 0 86388 313 2

Dedication

To all the older people who have shared their personal stories with me.

Special thanks to Frank for his patient encouragement throughout the writing process, and to the many friends who have shown ongoing interest and encouragement in the project.

Contents

Tables

Figures

Handouts

Sample Forms

Acknowledgements

It has only been possible to write this book because of my work with older people, first as a field social worker and more recently as a reminiscence worker. Being privy to the memories, thoughts and feelings of older people has been a great privilege and a constant learning experience.

In compiling this book I have incorporated my knowledge and experience of reminiscence work with older people. I have also studied the views and findings of other practitioners and researchers, in order to provide information on the theory of reminiscence work, and practical ideas on how to initiate and maintain this area of work.

The stories of individuals included in the book, which have been heavily disguised to ensure anonymity, are based on either my own work with older people, or the experiences of carers of older people shared with me in my role of reminiscence skills trainer.

I have been encouraged and supported in developing my reminiscence practice by Annis Tombs and Chris Franklin of Warwickshire Social Services.

Preface – *How to use this Handbook*

The information, thinking points and training activities included in this reminiscence handbook are designed to enhance carers' understanding, valuing and confidence in the process of reminiscence work with older people. The handbook provides a practical guide to initiating sensitive reminiscence work with individuals and small groups by promoting:

- An understanding of the term 'reminiscence work'
- Knowledge of the different forms of reminiscing
- An appreciation of the value of reminiscing to older people and their carers
- Increased valuing by carers of their own experiences, and of how the past has links with the present and future
- An understanding of the process of reminiscing
- Awareness of the skills, attitudes and values that promote positive reminiscing
- Understanding of how older people experience grief, and the role loss plays in the reminiscence process
- Increased empathy for older people by highlighting the complex and unique paths individuals have followed in becoming who they are today
- Skills for initiating and maintaining reminiscence work with individuals and small groups.

This book is designed to be used mainly by two groups of people:

1. *Carers* of older people in residential and nursing homes, hospitals and day-care centres, and carers in the community, for whom the information, thinking points and training activities will cover all aspects of the training needs of individuals wishing to develop one-to-one or group reminiscence work.

   Each training activity in this handbook can be used as the basis for a weekly workshop, to progressively build up knowledge, understanding and skills. Alternatively, individual activities may be combined to form a one- or two-day workshop.

Throughout the text, a number of the thinking points and training activities provide the opportunity for carers to experience, first-hand, how it feels to reminisce. In this way, carers are able to gain greater insight into the process and value of reminiscing.

2 *Independent trainers* working in the area of health and social care issues could use the activities to build one- or two-day workshops in reminiscence skills training. Additionally, many of the training activities would be appropriate to incorporate in courses covering issues such as developing person-centred care of older people; the role of bereavement and loss in older people's lives; and one-to-one and groupwork communication skills.

Introduction

That vivid present of theirs, how faint it grows! The past is only the present become invisible and mute and because it is invisible its memorial glances and murmurs are infinitely precious. MARY WEBB, *Precious Bane*

HOW I DISCOVERED REMINISCENCE

If this workbook is able to communicate even a little of the potential liveliness and creativity of reminiscence work waiting to be experienced by older people and their carers, it will be a success.

For me, reminiscence work came as a breath of fresh air after many years as a local authority social worker: it was stimulating to have the time as a sessional reminiscence worker to listen, to absorb and enjoy older people's histories. Reminiscence work provided an opportunity to combine an interest in social history with previous training in counselling, bereavement and loss, and groupwork skills.

The process of reminiscence work with older people can be addictive and absorbing. The enjoyment, stimulation and validation gained by the majority of older people from reminiscing makes it in turn a very rewarding experience for carers.

In looking to develop or extend personal knowledge of reminiscence work with older people, you may be a carer in a residential or nursing home, hospital or day setting for older people. Alternatively, you may have developed interest in the work as a carer of a relative, or as a voluntary visitor in the community. Whatever your role as a carer, and previous experience of reminiscence work, the information and training activities in this handbook will provide a practical guide to developing understanding and skills in this area of work with older people.

The process of reminiscing provides a varied, creative and absorbing means of communicating with individuals. It establishes communication links that are based on recalling the past, while bringing meaning, congruence and enjoyment to older people in the present. Carers who initiate reminiscence work with an older person begin the process of illuminating that individual's past: from the shared highlights of a life grows a greater awareness of an intricate and unique history. Insight is developed into the events that have moulded the individuals of today. Information gained through reminiscence work also provides a powerful reminder to carers that older people have passed through the same life stages that they have experienced, or will experience during their lives.

BREAKING DOWN BARRIERS

The realisation that there are common experiences transcending generations helps to break down barriers between older people and their carers. Reminiscence work provides opportunities for both carers and older people to grow and be enlivened by the process.

The individuality of older people is clearly highlighted through their recall of unique and revealing histories. This illuminating process of sharing through reminiscence work challenges set, and often limiting, expectations about how older people react and what they want from life. Equally helpful in avoiding restricting stereotyping is the willingness to become more aware of personal and societal attitudes to ageing attitudes that inevitably influence care patterns.

THINKING POINT

To become more aware of your thoughts about being older spend a few moments thinking about how you feel life should be for older people. Do you view later life as a time for quietness and the avoidance of new experiences? Or do you believe that everyone continues to learn, change and grow throughout life; and that carers have a role to play in providing opportunities for older people to continue to retain their interests and sociability?

Older people need to be physically safe and warm, and have a comfortable environment to live in. Having the opportunity to develop living patterns that make the world a familiar and secure place is crucial for their wellbeing. However, the challenge for carers is to promote both the physical, *and* the social and emotional aspirations of the older people they live or work with. To take up this challenge, carers need to offer opportunities to older people to enable them to maintain a feeling of purposefulness, a sense of individuality and self-esteem. Additionally, to enhance social and emotional care individuals need the opportunity to build meaningful relationships with carers that promote communication based on mutual liking and interest. Older people will be helped to flourish within this person-centred approach to care, with its commitment to acknowledging and maintaining individuality.

Reminiscence work has a major role to play within person-centred care practices by providing a tool to open up a two-way channel of communication between carer and older person. Reminiscing can be empowering in older people's lives: insights provided by the past can be indicators of the views, interests and preferences held by people in their daily lives in the present.

Kathy – a care assistant in a residential home – noticed how much Josie enjoyed reading novels. Josie told Kathy she had always loved reading as a child and that another pleasure had been going to the cinema for the Saturday matinee; she had not been for years. Kathy arranged for them both to go to the local cinema, much to Josie's delight.

In this example, Kathy was able to bring a past interest to life again for Josie, giving both of them pleasure and supporting a person-centred caring relationship in the present.

PAST, PRESENT AND FUTURE

If, as reminiscence workers, we listen well and respond with imagination and hope, individuals can feel valued for their unique experience of life, and we can help create continuity between who older people were and who they are today. Shared information about the past allows it to merge positively with the present and future.

Reminiscence work brings the past to life with a start. As workers, we need enthusiasm to hear individuals naming their past. Personal historical knowledge does not need to be great, but it is important to be able to communicate the value that the past has in all our lives. It is vital to be able to let individuals 'teach' us about what went before, and to be open to hearing their stories. Their journey may trigger personal memories of past events. To encourage positive reminiscence in others, carers need to be at ease with, and value, their own histories.

Reminiscence work can also reach out to individuals with dementia: the ability to recount personal stories from childhood and early adulthood is one of the last areas of memory to be affected by the eroding confusion of dementia.

Sensitive reminiscence work can help to build a bridge between a well-remembered and more secure past and the constantly changing present, a present where everyday life becomes increasingly confusing for people with dementia: an ever-growing maze to be lost in. Holding a conversation or carrying out a simple self-help task in the right order becomes daily more complex and difficult for individuals with dementia. Reminiscence work allows carers to break into this confusion by concentrating on areas of memory that are still intact, or less damaged, to communicate about the past, and to build relationships in the present.

Summary Points

Introduction to Reminiscence

- Reminiscence work is a creative communication tool, using the anchor of the past to build relationships in the present.
- Unique and diverse histories are highlighted and person-centred care practices supported through reminiscence work as carers are helped to understand the past experiences that have shaped the individuals of today.
- Reminiscence work can cut through the chaos of dementia to reach individuals via their memories of the past.
- Carers' views on the opportunities older people need to live fulfilling lives influence caring attitudes.
- The skills, values and attitudes needed for sensitive reminiscence work lie at the base of all good practice in the care of older people.

1 Reminiscence – *Origins, Characteristics and Value*

I do think that the present moment of the old contains all the past as well, which is vividly present as the present and makes it marvellously rich.
KATHLEEN MOORE, *Joyce Grenfell – An Invisible Friendship*

WHAT IS REMINISCING?

The creative, absorbing activity of reminiscing is available to everyone. As life is experienced memory develops, vocabulary grows and our reminiscence reservoir begins to fill.

When reminiscing, individuals remember the past: life stages, family events and relationships, hopes, dreams, losses and achievements, social and historical experiences. Remembrances may remain as private thoughts, or be shared on a one-to-one basis or in groups. Memories may be of a single event, or a series of linked or disconnected recollections.

Beginnings

The desire and need to pass down memories, wisdom and knowledge to future generations has always been strong across ages and cultures.

In earliest times information about events was preserved for those who followed through drawings and symbols. With the growth of the written word came scribes who recorded events for posterity. In traditional societies storytellers have long had a role in passing down myths and sacred stories essential to the continuation of the way of life of a particular culture.

Traditional songs also have a role to play in communicating across generations the happenings and mood of a certain time. For example, the patriotic songs of the First and Second World War are evocative of the mood and concerns of soldiers and their loved ones.

Up until the second half of the twentieth century, the inclination of older people to reminiscence was viewed negatively; it was believed that 'dwelling' on the past would inevitably lead to increased confusion and disconnection from the present.

By adopting this disparaging view of reminiscing, many professionals were echoing the view expressed by Aristotle (1995 translation) over 2,000 years previously. He observed the tendency in older people to remember the past and equated the process with a lack of hope:

> They live by memory rather than by hope for what is left to them of life is but little compared to the long past.

Increasingly since the 1970s, reminiscence work with older people has built up a reputation as being a 'hopeful' activity: acknowledged as offering a stimulating social experience. The beginning of a change of attitude to reminiscence work by social and health professionals is partly attributed to a paper written by a leading American psychiatrist, Robert Butler (1963), in which he strongly stated the view that reminiscing was a normal and healthy mental activity for older people to enter into.

There was an overwhelmingly positive response to Butler's endorsement of reminiscence work. Rose Dobroff, a social worker with older people in New York, writing in 1984, summed up the sense of liberation felt by carers in being encouraged to pursue reminiscence work:

> The old were free to remember, to regret, to look reflectively at the past and try to understand it. And we were free to listen and to treat rememberers and remembrances with the respect they deserved.

In Britain, reminiscence work in day and residential settings for older people was further promoted by the publication in 1981 of *Recall* by Help the Aged. This was a reminiscence aid that took the form of six sequences of audio tapes and slides. It provided a readily available resource for professionals working with older people to begin to explore reminiscence work. The idea had been initiated by Mick Kemp following his experience in the 1970s when, as a Department of Health and Social Security (DHSS) researcher, he noted that older people in residential homes unlike those living in the general community were not encouraged to talk about their past. Kemp, with other professionals, developed the aid to provide a focus for staff beginning the process of enabling older people in their care to remember the past.

Reminiscence work began to flourish in the early 1980s. Older people were increasingly invited to recall their histories, and carers were encouraged to listen, value and record the rich tapestries of shared memories.

Reminiscence today

An organisation active in promoting reminiscence work in Britain today is The Age Exchange Reminiscence Centre in Blackheath, London. Established in the late 1980s, it has become one of the key centres for training, drama and general work in reminiscence. As interest in the work grew across Europe, Age Exchange became the centre for the development of the European Reminiscence Network. The Network is currently involved in developing reminiscence projects, publishing the quarterly magazine *Reminiscence*, carrying out research and running conferences throughout Europe.

In Britain, as in other countries, at the start of the new millennium there has been a surge of general interest in recording, preserving and broadcasting individual oral histories of social and historical memories of the twentieth century. The Oral History Society is working to extend awareness about the value of preserving knowledge of the past through oral history records. The aim of the Society's conference in June 2001 was to bring together oral history projects from across Britain. The conference provided a national showcase for the work of community groups together with a forum to discuss common issues around oral history work.

In the USA and Australia, reminiscence work has experienced a steady increase since the 1990s. In the USA one of the organisations working to further good practice is The International Institute for Reminiscence and Life Review at the University of Wisconsin-Superior. The institute has set up Internet rooms where issues about reminiscence work can be discussed online with practitioners and researchers. The university has a digital library with access to articles, book reviews and other information about reminiscence and life review. Conferences are held biannually to review current international research and general developments in reminiscence work.

Throughout the USA, the Oral History Association and the Association of Personal Historians are working to promote the recall and preservation of memories through oral history. Both organisations forge links with the business sector in order to engage professionals, from many disciplines, in supporting individuals with the process of recalling and publication of their life histories. Memories are preserved in written form, on audio and videotapes and CD-ROMs.

In Australia, the value of the recall and preservation of oral history is also attracting growing recognition. In the year 2001, to mark the country's Centenary of Federation year, the Oral History Association organised a conference called 'Voices of a Twentieth Century Nation'. One of the themes of the conference was to consider how memories of the past, collected and preserved through oral histories, could help forge national identity in the present. The International Society for Folk Narrative Research also held a conference in 2001, which focused on the value of life history narratives in contributing to developing an understanding of current social issues connected with race, inter-generational relationships, and cultural and language differences.

In Britain, within residential and community settings for older people, the developing focus has been on group, one-to-one life review and life-story reminiscence work. Despite some growth in the promotion of reminiscence work in care settings, its use is still far from widespread. As a result, opportunities for promoting older people's sense of individuality are being lost when they are confronted with depersonalising group-living situations. Demands on staff time made by physical care routines, and low carer-to-client staff ratios are factors that are often attributed to the absence, or infrequency, of formal reminiscence work in care settings.

The reminiscence experience, with its emphasis on interaction between older people and their peers and carers, validates an individual's past through social exchanges in the present. Its potential to contribute to person-centred care patterns is great, providing an enriching way to access personal past history, which in turn offers insights into individuals' present actions and attitudes.

Increased longevity is resulting in ever-growing numbers of older people living independently in both the community and residential settings. (The Australian *National Health Strategy* (1991) predicted an increase of 103 percent between 1991 and 2001 in the numbers of older people aged over 85 years.) To ensure that older people continue to have quality, as well as quantity, of life there needs to be as great an emphasis on social and emotional 'health' as on physical wellbeing. The challenge to professional carers, voluntary workers and relatives is to consider how older people can be helped to continue to have the degree of purpose and sense of social belonging in their lives that is commensurate to their needs and wishes.

Research indicates that reminiscence work on a one-to-one basis and in small groups can contribute to the quality of life of older people: Tobin (1991) noted in his study that making the past come alive again, through reminiscence work with a sensitive listener, can be one of the main factors in continuing psychological wellbeing for older people. Individuals, Tobin believes, benefit greatly from revealing to others their past and present identities. Fielden (1990), focusing on small group reminiscence work in a sheltered housing complex, also concluded that the activity was beneficial to older people: a sense of increased wellbeing and enjoyment was observed in group members as a result of socialising with other residents.

Older people often develop an easily accessible and sharp memory focus on events from their more distant past. This heightened memory recall provides a rich source for reminiscence work. Conversely, they may find it increasingly difficult to make new memories due to short-term memory loss and/or decreasing opportunities for new experiences. Reminiscence, with its key to unlocking a past that may appear more purposeful, less lonely and inactive than the present, offers an appealing focus for rekindling the present.

REMINISCENCE IS NOT FOR EVERYONE

It is important, while acknowledging the significance of reminiscing in many older people's lives, to appreciate that its absence does not denote a failure to adapt positively to the process of ageing. Coleman (1991) emphasizes this point forcibly:

> Reminiscence can be a sign of successful ageing and high morale,
> and so can the absence of reminiscence.

It is essential to have a clear appreciation and acceptance of the reasons why reminiscing is not for everyone. From observations over a 10 year period, Coleman

(1986) identified differing responses to reminiscing among a group of older people living in sheltered housing schemes in London. He noted four distinct responses:

- Positive reminiscers enjoyed and valued memories recalled
- Negative reminiscers were distressed by painful memories
- Non-reminiscers did not see any value in dwelling on the past
- Non-reminiscers avoided memories of the past because of the feeling of loss that it provoked

Although there are many older people living in the community, or in residential and nursing settings, that enjoy reminiscing and the boost it gives to their self-esteem and coping capacities in the present, some older people are reluctant reminiscers, or actively avoid the experience.

For some individuals who do not want to reminiscence, there is no solace in memories: the comparison between their present lives, perhaps due to the limiting effects of disability or loss of a loved one, and the past, is too painful to contemplate. This may be an ongoing feeling, or a temporary reaction provoked by recent events, such as bereavement or a move to institutional care.

A minority of older people may be subject to recurring memories associated with one or a number of traumatic life incidents that provoke bitter, regretful and persistently distressing thoughts about their own or others' actions. Complicated responses to past bereavements or horrific war experiences are examples of events that may provoke ongoing traumatic reactions. These older people may openly reject being involved in reminiscence work, from a fear of being overwhelmed by their painful memories. However, the distress may be so great and close to the surface that it leaks into their daily lives as the offending memories, unprompted, are persistently and painfully recalled. In such instances, skilled counselling intervention is required, to allow sufficient time and expertise to help individuals, if possible, to resolve or to go some way towards resolving their feelings about the traumatic event.

A group of older people for whom reminiscence plays only a small, if any, role in their lives are those who feel that their present life is too full to spend time looking back. Such people are those who retain their health and live independently in the community. For them, there remain opportunities to enjoy new experiences, retain their freedom and continue to pursue past and new interests.

THINKING POINT

Do you know an older person who shows a negative response to reminiscing? Have they shared with you the reasons why remembering does not appeal to them?

Individuals who feel reluctant to reminisce in a group may be more receptive to one-to-one sensitive life-review reminiscence work, which provides the opportunity for them to give vent to painful feelings from the past or present, and revisit events in an attempt to make sense of what happened.

REMINISCENCE AND BEREAVEMENT

Bereavement reminiscence has a major role to play in helping older people to cope with loss. One-to-one work provides the opportunity to recall the circumstances of past and recent deaths; to express painful feelings provoked by the loss; remember the loved one and share memories; and to express any confusing or disturbing thoughts about the loss. The need to talk about the deceased and the death is normal, and a number of regular sessions may be required before there is less intensity and more acceptance by the bereaved person. This form of one-to-one bereavement reminiscence work helps older people gain relief through the expression of natural distress in response to a changed and painful situation.

Giving up a permanent home to move into a care setting is a loss of independence, familiarity and freedom. It too is a bereavement, capable of provoking many of the feelings and thoughts normally associated with reactions to a death.

Through sensitive bereavement reminiscence work, older people may be helped to release their natural bereavement feelings, and so move through the aching hurt of loss and find some pleasure in remembrance of a past that contained a loved one and/or a more independent way of living. In reaching some degree of reconciliation with the past, the present and future may become more tolerable and worthwhile.

This topic will be developed in Chapter 7 – 'Promoting One-to-One Reminiscence Work'.

REFLECTING ON THE PAST AND PRESENT

Within the reminiscence process, it is important to avoid over-emphasising the role of the past, to the exclusion of the present, in older people's lives. Over-emphasis may result in a lack of awareness in carers as to the impact that events in the daily life of older people have on influencing their social, emotional and physical wellbeing.

Harris and Hopkins (1995) highlight the possibility that reminiscence can minimise the credibility and attention carers give to the current issues in older people's daily lives: for very positive and respectful reasons, carers within the reminiscence process often accord older people the role of being 'all-knowing' about the past. Harris and Hopkins point out that casting older people in this 'sage role' has a stereotyping effect, creating a preoccupation with the past and a resultant diminution of emphasis on the daily fabric of individuals' lives.

The preoccupation with the 'all-knowing' role of older people need not be a drawback in the reminiscence process, if information gained or highlighted is used constructively to enliven and improve the current lives of older people. Institutions can be humanised by meeting as many personal preferences as possible; by encouraging resumption of past interests; and by developing social activities based on increased knowledge of residents' past skills and interests. Furthermore, believing generally in the value that the past has to play in influencing individuals' present lives does not preclude older people and/or their carers from fighting against age-related discriminatory practice in the present. In addition reminiscence, with its ability to strengthen the concept of self, plays a role in helping older people have the confidence to counter and overcome negative aspects of their present lives.

Table 1 summarises the characteristics of reminiscence work, which will be developed in this and later chapters of this handbook.

Table 1 · **SUMMARY OF THE KEY CHARACTERISTICS OF REMINISCENCE WORK**

Forms of reminiscing	◆ Solitary, one-to-one or group-based. ◆ Spontaneous and informal or structured and planned; life review and life-story work or groupwork. ◆ Individuals may enjoy one or all forms of reminiscing. ◆ One-to-one work is appropriate for individuals sharing bereavement reminiscences or compiling memories books. ◆ Not everyone wants to reminiscence: contrast between past and present may be too painful; certain events may provoke too many hurtful memories to recall.
Recall	◆ Using triggers that appeal to one or more different senses – smell, sight, hearing, touch and taste – prompt remembering. ◆ The more specific and personal a trigger, the greater its potential for prompting memories. ◆ Artefacts, music, drawing, miming and individuals taking part in traditional domestic tasks all prompt memories. ◆ Sharing one memory can set off a reminiscence chain on the same or different subjects. ◆ Memories are vivid and enable individuals to be transported back to another time. ◆ Not all recollections are happy: life is a mixture of happy, sad and ordinary times. ◆ Great pleasure is obtained from getting in touch with memories not previously recalled.
Timings	◆ Older people potentially have a lifetime of experience to share; the process cannot be hurried. Allowing sufficient time for individual and group sessions acknowledges the value of the memories being shared. ◆ Be prepared to give time to respond to prompts, rephrasing questions if necessary.
Self-worth	◆ Sharing the map of our lives with all of its major routes, cul-de-sacs, diversions and minor roads of experience, helps to maintain and develop feelings of being valued. ◆ Individuals, by making their history come alive, use the past to communicate in the present; caring and peer relationships are enhanced. ◆ Information gained through reminiscence can indicate how patterns of care can be more person-centred.

The different forms that reminiscence work can take for an individual are illustrated by the reminiscence route taken by one older person, Annie (see case study below).

Annie, who is 84, moved to her residential home two years ago following a long illness. Annie had worked in the local manufacturing industry and all her life had lived within two miles of the home. She has four children, all now aged over 60 years.

Annie regularly talked of the pleasure gained in the time she spent in the evenings in *solitary reminiscing.* This involved visualising the local area and remembering the houses and streets where she had lived:

'When I'm sitting quietly I often take a "walk" down my old street, remembering who lived where and what each shop sold. It is such a relaxing thing to do.', she said.

Annie was particularly close to one carer at the home who knew her daughters. During brief chats with the carer Annie had the opportunity to share her memories in *spontaneous, informal one-to-one reminiscing.* Often news about present-day happenings in the neighbourhood triggered Annie to recollect how she and her family had lived in the past. Recall during these conversations was sometimes restricted to one set of memories related directly to the carer's comments; at other times a memory chain would be stimulated that was unconnected to the original conversation. One memory would lead to another, vividly recreating parts of Annie's past for herself and her carer.

Annie also attended a *reminiscence group* for six sessions with a small number of other residents. The group offered the opportunity to take part in a *formal, structured reminiscence* experience aimed at stimulating the recall and sharing of personal experience. Each session had a theme to encourage initial conversation. Annie particularly enjoyed the session on clothing. The artefacts including old hats and gloves were evocative triggers for Annie, reminding her in particular of her grandmother's love of gloves. She recalled how her grandmother had many pairs, ranging from everyday cotton ones to fancy elbow-length French gloves, the latter being worn only for weddings and other special occasions.

Annie had been greatly influenced by her grandmother who was a colourful and forceful character in her life. Later on, she developed the memories triggered in this group reminiscence in a memories book. This involved *one-to-one reminiscence* work spending an hour a week for four sessions during which Annie shared many memories of her life. One of the sessions involved a drive out to take photographs of Annie's childhood home and places where she and her parents had worked. Annie's memories were recorded with photographs and other items referring to her life to form a memories book.

During the compilation of the book, Annie had the opportunity to look back over parts of her life, and her experiences of childhood, marriage, work, and now life in a residential home. She touched on painful emotions surrounding the death of parents and siblings, and how difficult it was to come to terms with the loss of independence due to her disability.

> This evaluation of life, which may include going over happy and sad events, coping with living with disability and looking at feelings about the individual's own death, is termed *life review*. This form of reminiscence work may involve the individual recalling a number of events or can be restricted to one memory that was particularly upsetting or changed the individual's life dramatically.
>
> Annie enjoyed taking part in all the different forms of reminiscing. She often spoke of how relaxing and absorbing she found it to talk about the past, either in a one-to-one or group situation.

This handbook will largely focus on the skills and issues involved in initiating and maintaining formal, structured reminiscence work in small groups and on a one-to-one basis. The emphasis in one-to-one work will be on how to help older people take part in life review work, and compile memories books.

THE VALUE OF PROMOTING REMINISCENCE WORK

This book is for carers looking to introduce or develop reminiscence work with older people. Therefore, the emphasis will be primarily on considering the value of the activity for older people. However, it is important and encouraging to realise the satisfaction that being involved in reminiscence activities can hold for carers too. Some of the benefits that older people and their carers can gain through reminiscence work are examined below.

Support at times of change

One of the major social and emotional challenges faced by older people is a move to residential living, a challenge that is often confronted when individuals are at their most vulnerable. Emotional and physical resources may be low, due to increasing physical and/or mental health difficulties, perhaps coupled with the pain of loss due to the death of a partner or other supportive relative. At this time of distress and loss, older people have to adapt to living in a new environment with a large number of strangers.

Reminiscence work offers a way of breaking through the initial anonymity of moving into residential care, with its power of enabling carers to build up a picture of individuals' lives, past and present. Additionally, at this time of loss and change, reminiscence work offers an opportunity for sharing bereavement reminiscence about the death of loved ones and/or the loss of a familiar way of life.

Thinking Point

To experience a little of the feeling that older people have when confronted with the need to move to sheltered or residential accommodation, spend a few moments looking around your home. Think about how many objects you would have to leave behind if tomorrow you moved to residential care. What feelings do you experience, just thinking about leaving your present home with limited possessions?

Relationship-building

Many older people feel restricted and resentful when faced with major changes to their daily routines, due to an increased dependence on others. Reduced ability in self-care may result in the need for day-care, or a permanent move to a sheltered or residential setting. Older people in these situations have to cope with new regimes, restrictions of choice, and less personal space than at any other time in their lives. Reminiscence has a role to play in helping them to feel at ease with new surroundings and people. It offers an invaluable way of building reciprocal relationships with carers and peers. The reminiscence process itself emphasizes the past, but is an activity based on communicating in the present.

A sensitive reminiscence atmosphere can generate feelings of trust, self-esteem and purposefulness in older people. Carers develop a greater sense of the whole person by becoming aware of the route older people have taken in reaching where, and who they are in the present. Revealing the intricacies of older people's past lives offers insights into present attitudes, needs and preferences. The awareness created by such insights fosters positive person-centred care patterns.

Reminiscence work can be effective in easing the transition of new residents to care settings: feelings of strangeness and isolation can be lessened as barriers are broken down through the sharing of common experiences with peers. Carers, through the reminiscence process, can promote communication by making links between individuals who have similar interests, or who have lived and worked in the same area.

Active not passive

All reminiscence work promotes the active involvement of older people; indeed, without their commitment it becomes a lifeless activity. The emphasis in reminiscence on the active involvement of older people shifts the focus of attention for carers, for a time, from the demands of physical dependence needs to emotional and social needs. As a result, older people are no longer viewed as dependent individuals, passively waiting to be helped, but as active and essential contributors to a social process.

Faith Gibson (1989) supports the view that reminiscence work offers a challenge to the traditionally held expectations of care priorities, where the primary emphasis is on physical care routines.

> People, and listening to people, may become more important than maintaining present policies and prevailing regimes where the first priority is physical care.

Carers who have the opportunity, through reminiscence work, to learn more about the older people they support show increased empathy towards them; relationships improve throughout the caring process.

Older people are actively empowered by the reminiscence process, as illustrated by Ken's comments to the leader of his memories group:

> We have so much to tell you about the past, of times you cannot imagine; we can teach you so much.

For a short time in reminiscence groups or one-to-one work, older people, like Ken, can redress the imbalance within the caring role: no longer mere passive receptacles of help. They are actively needed and valued by carers to entertain and inform others.

THINKING POINT

Can you think of an older person you have cared for who has taken pleasure, as Ken did, in feeling empowered within the caring relationship?

What was the situation? How did you react to this?

Pleasurable experience

Reminiscence work provides a valuable experience for older people because of the pleasure that many gain from the activity. It offers a stimulating, absorbing, social experience within a group setting or on a one-to-one basis. For the majority of older people, it provides a welcome addition to the daily routine. Carers are seen in a new light as interested and valuing listeners, able to promote the sharing of a distant past that returns to life for a time.

As mentioned above, not everyone wishes to recall their past. Additionally reminiscence activities may appeal to individuals at certain times, but not at others. For example, an older person may reject the experience when they are pre-occupied with health or other concerns, but may be willing to join in when such concerns are resolved or eased. It is important that individuals understand that an initial refusal does not preclude them from taking part on another occasion.

Individuals gain enjoyment from different forms of reminiscence work in various ways, as illustrated by the case of Winnie.

> Winnie attended a number of group reminiscence sessions, but was very reluctant to share her past with her peers. However, she enjoyed listening to others and the change of scene that the activity provided.
>
> One day Winnie was asked if she would enjoy completing a memories book (life-story book). She agreed, and in one-to-one sessions readily shared memories, especially about her young adulthood.
>
> One memory in particular would bring forth chuckles and evident pleasure in recall:
>
>> 'In my lunch hour I would often go to Lewis' department store in the city centre where they had a pianist playing in the restaurant. I would talk to the pianist in the interval and told her on one occasion that I played the piano at a high-grade level. The next day she asked me to stand in for her for 10 minutes whilst she nipped out on an errand, which I did. No-one seemed to notice any difference and I was really pleased with myself.'
>
> Winnie was animated recalling this memory and others, in a one-to-one reminiscence session. The pleasure she gained from actively sharing memories in one-to-one reminiscence contrasted sharply to the quieter listening experience in a group setting. For Winnie, both were acknowledged as enjoyable activities, offering an interesting variation to her normal routine.

Reaching into dementia

Reminiscence work with people with dementia is a hopeful, positive way of relating to individuals increasingly lost in the baffling maze of everyday life. It provides the opportunity for meaningful and specific communication about the past in the present. Reminiscence work enables carers to appreciate and utilise those skills and long-term memory areas that remain for the individual with dementia. It offers a counter to carers' feelings of being overwhelmed and powerless as they confront the changes and losses experienced by individuals with dementia.

An individual's earliest memories and skill acquisitions are the last to be lost to dementia. Reminiscence work, with its emphasis on the sharing of personal stories, capitalises on these remaining areas of memory. Additionally, when the ability to recall even early life finally succumbs to dementia, information gained previously through the reminiscence process can be returned to the individual, thus helping to prolong a sense of identity.

Older people with dementia retain enjoyment in life and can continue to gain pleasure-in-the-moment. Reminiscence work is able to offer such pleasure in the moment: enjoyment and stimulation can be experienced, particularly if triggers are specific to the individual's life.

Maintaining a sense of identity

Reminiscence work fosters a continuing sense of self by providing space for older people's personal stories to be acknowledged, valued and remembered. Reminiscence activities offer a counter to the anonymity of residential settings. By being encouraged to share personal histories, older people feel they are still significant, and are able to retain social connections and be valued for their unique experiences. In reclaiming and acknowledging the past, older people are reminded of the potential power of their own voice in the present.

Group, or one-to-one reminiscence work with individuals from under-represented ethnic minority groups within a care setting helps to maintain and develop both individual and group cultural identities. Long-held values are reaffirmed for older people through the sensitive interest and respect shown by carers in the traditions and beliefs of minority cultures.

Stanley Hamilton, quoted in the *Reminiscence Magazine*, illustrates an example of the impact that reaffirming past cultural traditions can have on older people and their carers:

> I remember on one occasion a mid-winter ritual using candles. As I held out a candle to one woman, she began to intone the Jewish Sabbath prayer. This was a totally unexpected moment with great power and beauty, which restored to her a lost part of her past life.

Similar shared moments between carers and older people nurture communication and increase empathy for individuals who have grown old outside their country of origin.

Additionally, insights and information gained by carers during the reminiscence process can be beneficial in planning more sensitive programmes of care for older people from minority groups.

Promoting life-review

Sensitive, empathetic one-to-one life-review reminiscence work is a process that aims to promote reflection on, and expression of, positive and negative feelings about past events in order to help individuals reach reconciliation with the past. In life, everyone encounters difficulties, losses, high and low points. Many older people inevitably feel regret, possibly guilt, about their role in certain situations and events. For older people, the past often takes on a sharp, intense focus; there may be the need to replay memories in an attempt to understand and accept past events.

Older people, through life-review reminiscence work, are helped to make their peace with the past by sharing the impact of important life events. American gerontologists Gray Soltys and Grudzen (2000), in their consideration of the role of reminiscence in the lives of older people observe that a growing sense of mortality commonly provokes 'evaluative reminiscing'. They discuss an example of evaluative reminiscing:

> Mr J, an older man dying of cancer, despite extensive reminiscing was unable to let go of the guilt he felt towards his ex-wife and daughters. Mr J only obtained release from his past once his ex-wife had visited and the couple were able to discuss their life together. Mr J's ex-wife expressed forgiveness for his past actions and, released from his guilt, Mr J died only hours later.

Equally, the death of close family and friends in the present can result in intense feelings of loss, when pain from unresolved past bereavements is intermingled with current grief.

Sensitive, one-to-one life-review work helps to promote the positive view that life is a continuous flow of experiences with understanding gained from the past enhancing coping capacities in the present.

Life-review work can also valuably provide the opportunity to name and celebrate life's satisfactions: achievements and good fortune can be recalled and shared. In life-review sessions, older people often repeat expressions that sum up the pleasure they have experienced in their lives:

> Susie, almost 90, utilised life-review time as a channel to happily restate a positive summary of the past relationships in her life. Her words suggest a strong satisfaction in how her life had been lived:
>
> > 'I had a wonderful mom and dad. A wonderful husband, John, and two caring daughters. Who could ask for more?'

Overall gains for both the carer and older person, from taking part in a life-review process, include increased trust and an enhanced sense of connection within the caring relationship.

Summary Points

Origins, Characteristics and Value of Reminiscence

- Reminiscing is the process in which individuals recall and share memories of the past.
- Older people enjoy reminiscing as a solitary experience, in a one-to-one situation, and in small groups.
- Not all recollections are happy; unresolved and painful memories may be expressed in reminiscence work.
- Reminiscence work is beneficial both to carers and older people, enhancing relationships through a greater understanding and sharing of the past.
- The individuality of older people shines through in reminiscence work, countering stereotypical views.
- Reminiscence validates individuals' past lives, and builds bridges between the past and present.
- Reminiscence activities are fun, entertaining and relaxing for older people and their carers.
- The impact of dementia may be lessened by the ability of reminiscence work to capitalise on remaining memory areas, and to offer valuable 'pleasure-in-the-moment' experiences.

2 Promoting Reminiscence

I have found it enriching to open channels whereby others can communicate their feelings, their private perceptual worlds, to me.
CARL ROGERS, *A Therapist's View of Psychotherapy – On Becoming a Person*

This chapter highlights the skills, knowledge and attitudes needed by carers to promote sensitive reminiscence work.

Carers' practice in their work with older people is dependent on a complex mixture of personal attributes, life experience, client-related skills and knowledge base, and a personal and organisational view of the needs and rights of older people.

It is important that carers, before initiating reminiscence work, acknowledge and respect certain key attitudes based on valuing older people's histories and the uniqueness of all individuals. These core attitudes indicate a belief in the need to preserve the 'personhood' of individuals. The acquisition of relevant skills and knowledge needed to develop positive reminiscence work is achieved through training, reading, practise, supervision and sharing experiences with colleagues and supervisors, as shown in Table 2.

Table 2 · **KEY COMPONENTS IN DEVELOPING POSITIVE REMINISCENCE WORK**

Skills	**Knowledge**	**Attitudes**
Active listening skills to respond sensitively to verbal and non-verbal communication.	Group processes: to understand the roles individuals play in groups, and how to promote group identity.	Promoting 'personhood': acknowledging and respecting the uniqueness of individuals.
To be empathetic: to experience another's world, without losing the sense of self.	Bereavement process: to be able to recognise normal and complicated responses to loss situations.	Valuing of older people's histories, and enjoying being 'taught' about the past.
To take part in reminiscence 'research': to increase background knowledge of individuals.	To find out about different cultural and religious norms.	To acknowledge the role of older people's past in their present lives.
To recognise when referral to an outside agency for specialist support is appropriate.	To be self-aware about personal feelings towards loss, so that we can really 'hear' others.	To promote older people in taking an active, not passive role socially.

Two of the main areas involved in the promotion of positive reminiscence work are the use of effective listening and groupwork skills. The following is an exploration of the role played by these two main elements of successful reminiscence work.

EFFECTIVE LISTENING SKILLS

Familiarity with the need to listen and respond in personal and professional communications may lead to an undervaluing of the role this skill area plays in promoting sensitive reminiscence work. During reminiscence activities, carers are faced with a variety of challenges in terms of communicating effectively, including handling emotion in life-review work; bringing harmony to a discordant group; and decoding the confusion of dementia using verbal and non-verbal messages as clues to meaning and needs.

THINKING POINT

To begin to highlight the skills of effective listening, reflect on the last occasion you felt really listened to, following which you recall feeling more at ease, accepted and understood. Think about how the person responded verbally and non-verbally to you in order to promote this feeling of really being listened to.

Listening sensitively involves the need to 'tune in' to individuals, in order to both hear the spoken message and pick up on emotions and meanings conveyed by non-verbal 'language'. It is possible to undervalue the messages sent and received through non-verbal clues, including facial expressions, eye-contact and gestures. Non-verbal messages play a major role in all communication. Research by Albert Mehrabian (1972) emphatically confirmed the impact of non-verbal communication. In his findings, only 7 per cent of the emotional meaning of messages was transmitted purely by verbal 'language'; 38 per cent was communicated by tone and voice intonation; while 55 per cent of the emotional content of messages was received through non-verbal cues.

To respond effectively, attitudes, words and non-verbal responses need to communicate understanding and acceptance of an individual's thoughts and feelings. Effective listeners are particularly skilled in communicating empathy for individuals. Empathy grows from the ability to sense how others experience their world. The skill of expressing empathy develops from listening well, and willingness to be alongside individuals as they explore their personal situation. Empathy, although communicated through responses and attitudes, is not simply a technique used in effective listening but a way 'of being' in relation to others, as illustrated in Table 3.

Table 3 · LEARNING HOW TO 'TUNE IN' VERBALLY AND NON-VERBALLY

Non-Verbally

- Overcoming personal distractions, sitting with an open posture at the same level as the individual.
- Illustrating close attention and concern by maintaining eye contact, without staring.
- Appropriate nods and facial expressions to communicate acceptance and understanding.
- Promotion of the expression of feelings without interruptions.
- Accepting silences without rushing in to fill the space.

Verbally

- Being clear about the time available to talk together.
- Recognising and acknowledge feelings expressed to communicate empathy: being alongside an individual in their world for a time.
- Showing interest and concern with supportive comments, such as 'Yes, I can see how hard that must have been for you.' Or, 'It sounds as if that was very difficult for you.'
- Use of open-ended questions to encourage sharing of thoughts and feelings, such as 'How did his words make you react?'; 'What were your feelings when that happened?'; 'How do you think you will cope now it has happened?'
- Avoiding attempts to minimise feelings with platitudes or comfort that may prevent the expression of painful feelings; using prompting questions to give individuals an opportunity to explore feelings further, for example: 'That sounds a painful time for you, would it help to say some more about how you felt at that point?'
- Valuing what has been shared as sessions finish.
- Helping individuals to 'come back' to present time at the end of sessions with references to the here and now.

Figure 1 shows the Chinese characters that make up the verb 'to listen'. It succinctly highlights the complex combination of senses and feelings utilised in the art of responsive listening.

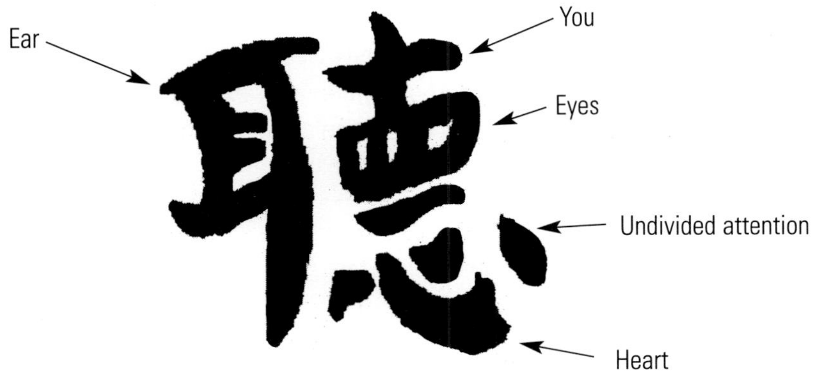

Figure 1 The Chinese characters that make up the verb 'to listen'

By employing verbal and non-verbal communication skills, listeners illustrate their willingness to hear distress without rushing in with quick reassurances that block expression of feelings. Also communicated is readiness on the listener's part to be empathetic and accepting.

When communicating with older people with dementia, skills are required in responding to communications that do not always have a literal meaning, and/or illustrate extreme short-term memory loss. Additionally, communications may include repetitious requests connected with demands to see deceased relatives or return to a past home. Communicating with a person with dementia demands enhanced listening and responding skills, detailed knowledge of the individual's background, and the willingness to build on interests, abilities and memory areas that remain (see Chapter 5, 'Reminiscence Work and the Challenge of Dementia'). Another specialised area of communication is in helping older people with issues and feelings that accompany loss (see Chapter 7, 'Promoting One-to-One Reminiscence Work').

The following case studies will aid understanding about the effective listening and responding skills described above. They show the kinds of comments often expressed by older people during reminiscence work, and suggest some of the feelings and thoughts that may motivate such comments. Ideas about ways of responding are also given.

Example One

Ivy was 91 years old. She had lived alone in a bungalow since her husband's death five years before, but for the last two years she had had regular falls the last of which resulted in a fractured hip. Following her recovery Ivy had not returned home, but had moved to residential care from hospital. Ivy's daughter had cleared the bungalow without wanting to worry her mother about choosing which possessions she kept or sold. As a result, Ivy's room in the home was bare, with little of her own furniture.

Ivy commented to her key worker, Diane, a few weeks after her admission: 'I miss my bungalow so much, it is as if that part of my life never existed, all my things have gone, I didn't even see my home for one last time. I can't get used to being here. What is the point of it all?'

What do you sense are the feelings conveyed by Ivy's words?

Possible feelings: sadness, emptiness, loneliness.

Possible response:

> 'Ivy, you sound very sad and lonely. Giving up your bungalow, without an opportunity to say goodbye, has made you feel as if part of your past has been lost. It is hard for you to adjust to living with lots of strangers and now you wonder what it has all been for.'

In her response, Diane has been able to reflect back to Ivy some of the feelings she expressed. In this way Diane is 'tuning in' to Ivy and acknowledging her pain. This response is verbally empathetic, helping Ivy to feel Diane understands and is able to accept her feelings.

An alternative response would be to reflect back just one of the feelings Diane sensed in Ivy's words:

> 'Ivy, life sounds sad and empty at the moment.' At this point, Diane could perhaps touch Ivy's hand, to acknowledge her distress.

Both of the responses would encourage Ivy to feel understood, and to go on sharing her feelings with Diane, perhaps expressing any feelings she had about her daughter clearing the bungalow without her involvement. By creating an effective listening atmosphere in which Ivy feels able to share her feelings, Diane is not making any judgements about Ivy or her daughter, but is 'tuning in' to Ivy's need to express and understand her emotions about the major adjustment she is facing on moving into residential care.

Example Two

George is 90 and has lived in a residential home for three years. He is a widower with two sons. He has regular contact with one son, Peter, and his family. He has not seen his other son, David, for 10 years. Joan, a carer, had been talking to George about his family. George suddenly looked sad, telling Joan that during a recent visit Peter had told him that his other son David was seriously ill.

'I would really like to go to see David', said George. 'But we had a row 10 years ago about his divorce, and the new woman he was living with. His mom and me thought David had been very unfair to his wife. She was a grand girl and he had let her down. I haven't seen David since the row and miss him so much. What shall I do?'

What feelings do you sense behind George's words?

Possible feelings: fear, pride, sadness, confusion.

Possible response:

> 'George you sound very worried about David. You feel he was wrong all those years ago but not seeing him for so long has made you sad and lonely. You are not sure what to do about visiting David. Would seeing David make you feel easier, whatever his reaction to you was?'

Joan's response acknowledges past and present feelings about George's situation. She has been able to reflect back to George both the meaning in his words, and the sense of his underlying feelings. Joan is not telling George what to do about visiting his son, but encouraging him to think more about the situation in order to reach his own conclusions.

An alternative response would be to focus on George's very positive feelings about seeing his son:

> 'George you speak of being unsure about seeing David because of the past but you looked and sounded so definite when you said you really wanted to see him again. Your need to see David again sounded stronger than your fears, is that how it feels?'

This response again 'tunes in' to spoken and unspoken feelings, and illustrates how well Joan is listening and being alongside George. Joan is not making a judgement about whether or not George should see his son again, but is summing up the verbal and non-verbal messages he is giving about what he wants to do. Additionally, with her last probing question, Joan offers an opportunity for George to explore his thoughts further. Again, the emphasis is on George making his own decision about contact with David.

BARRIERS TO EFFECTIVE LISTENING

It is important to be aware that internal and external distractions can be a barrier to effective listening in one-to-one or group reminiscence sessions. Distractions may be present in the general physical environment, or may arise from the listener's personal attitudes or concerns. Table 4 summarises possible external distractions; Table 5 focuses on possible internal distractions.

Table 4 · **EXTERNAL DISTRACTIONS TO EFFECTIVE LISTENING**

Noise	**Outdoors** ◆ Roadworks, building sites, heavy traffic. **Indoors:** ◆ Television, music, other people's conversation, telephones, bleepers.
Environment	◆ Uncomfortable seating or room temperature.
Other tasks	◆ Conflicting demands, including phone calls or queries.

Table 5 · INTERNAL DISTRACTIONS TO EFFECTIVE LISTENING

Inattentive behaviour	◆ Lack of eye contact, fidgeting, sitting at a distance or using furniture as a barrier.
Blocking expression	◆ Actively blocking individuals in their expression of thoughts and feelings. ◆ Exhibiting facial expressions that could be viewed as judgemental or severe, such as frowning or raising eyebrows.
Personal attitudes	◆ Holding set views on how others should live their lives, which may result in shocked or judgemental responses to individuals. ◆ Having strong prejudicial views against groups of people, resulting in dislike and fearful responses. ◆ Showing a strong need to give advice, or rush in with reassurance preventing individuals reaching their own solutions to difficulties or fully expressing troubled feelings.
Personal feelings	◆ Tired and overwhelmed from listening to other difficulties. ◆ Irritation and impatience with another's comments or behaviour: listening to constant repetition can be demanding and exhausting at times. ◆ Fears about the future of loved ones and the recall of personal past losses may be stimulated when listening to others. ◆ Awareness and acceptance of personal feelings about past losses helps in the ability to listen and respond well to others in loss situations.

THINKING POINT

Can you recall a time recently when you have been aware of external or internal distractions preventing you from listening well to someone? How did you overcome these distractions?

The skill of communicating effectively is a complex and demanding one. Within the reminiscence process effective listening can open informative, rewarding and valuable communication links with individuals. Reminiscence work with older people inevitably creates listening situations where carers need to be prepared to hear and respond to strong emotions about past and present lives. If carers are able to listen and respond with attention, empathy and genuine respect, the older person will feel understood, accepted and valued.

Additionally, it is essential for carers to acknowledge when available time and skills do not match the complexity of the issues, or depth of feeling expressed by older people. In such instances carers may be at a loss as to how to deal with the situation. This is the point at which referral to an outside agency for specialised counselling input may be appropriate. A minority of residential and nursing homes recognise the need for specialised skills in counselling when working with older people and employ counsellors on a sessional basis to deal with complex situations. This move is welcome, and will hopefully become more widespread in the future.

GROUPWORK

Groups are formed within a wide variety of contexts, to cover a multiplicity of activities, including self-help, consciousness-raising and therapy; social concern and political protest; educational and community initiatives. Groups are made up of collections of individuals with a shared sense of purpose, identity, aims and objectives. There are often definite criteria for membership of particular groups and ground rules to help members work together.

There are a large variety of models of groupwork and styles of leadership. The way (model) that reminiscence groups operate involves mutual sharing of memories on common or linked themes, from the distant or more recent past; memories may have a feeling as well as factual content. The skill in the leadership role is to promote a supportive, relaxed and caring atmosphere where memories are valued and individuals are enabled to make links with peers through common experiences, feelings and interests. In order to facilitate sensitive and supportive reminiscence groupwork group leaders need an understanding of how groups function generally.

Possessing knowledge and insight about how groups operate is valuable in understanding what is happening at any given time in group sessions. Reminiscence groups, in common with all kinds of groups, pass through stages in their development. Groupworkers Randall and Southgate (1980) believe that groups pass through four chronological stages in their development, which they term as 'nurturing', 'energising', 'peaking' and 'relaxing'. The Randall and Southgate model of the life of a group provides a valuable way of interpreting the process of group reminiscence sessions.

Nurturing stage

'Nuturing' is the term given to the initial stage in group formation by Randall and Southgate. In terms of reminiscence groups, this is the phase at the beginning of each session when the group needs to reform. As part of the 'nurturing' process, prior to the start of each weekly session, group leaders may need to encourage group members to attend. Encouragement may take the form of a recap about what format the group session takes; who else attends; duration and venue. Further 'nurturing' by leaders may include recalling for individuals what they enjoyed about attending the group in previous sessions. A typical conversation at this stage in group 'nurturing' may take the following form:

> 'Hello Mabel, I'm Joyce, the leader of the Memories Group you come to each Wednesday for about an hour. Last week we enjoyed your memories about your time in service as a maid. Would you like to come along with me to the Day Room for this week's session?'

The Randall and Southgate model describes this initial stage of 'nurturing' as a success if group members are given the space to say how they feel, and listen to others in a supportive way. As individuals gather together in the reforming phase of a reminiscence group session, information is shared about how members feel. Group members' comments may be directed at leaders during this initial regrouping stage. However, prompting individuals to talk to each other, offering reminders about names if necessary, helps to recreate feelings of a group identity in this 'nurturing' stage.

Energising stage

One of the ways in which the next stage in the group process that is termed 'energising' is achieved, is for the leader(s) to introduce an activity that builds on the renewed feeling of group identity fostered in the initial 'nurturing' stage. For example, a basket of artefacts could be passed around, with everyone being asked to select one item of interest. Individuals, in turn, are requested to say what they like about the selected item, or what it reminds them of. The leader(s), where possible, makes links between individuals who share similar memories or thoughts. In this way, the sense of group identity is increased. An example of the leader making a link between group members would be a response as follows:

> 'Helen and Vera you chose old tiles from the basket, recalling how they reminded you both of the design of your family open fire surround. It would be interesting to know if you both had to take a turn in black leading the grate.'

The Randall and Southgate model views the 'energising' stage as being a success if an accepting atmosphere is created in a group, with all members feeling able to express their thoughts easily. Promoting group activities that lead to the expression of memories and establishing links between individuals helps to attain this positive, creative 'energising' phase of the group process.

Peaking stage

The model describes the third phase in the group process as being the 'peak' stage. In the life of a reminiscence session, this phase can be clearly identified at the point when the group has been recalling memories for a period of time, creating a tangible feeling of group togetherness, sharing and general enjoyment. At this point in the session, group members often express surprise at how many memories have been recalled in a short time. The 'peak' stage in a group can also be achieved by accomplishing a task together: preparing and cooking a cake is one example. In this group task, members can be encouraged to take a turn in weighing and mixing or giving advice on how it would have been done in the past. Seeing, smelling and tasting the success of the group task creates a 'peak' in enjoyment for its members. The following comment is an illustration of the 'peak' enjoyment often experienced by members at this stage of the group process:

> 'It's ages since any of us did any cooking, but we've made a good job of the cake between us.'

Relaxing stage

After this 'peak' has been reached in the reminiscence session, the group enters the final 'relaxing' stage. Taking time over refreshments can facilitate this stage of the group process. During this period, group members and leader(s) can look back on the session, reminding each other about what was shared, and planning for the next meeting. At this concluding point in the group session, members are often surprised at how fast the time has gone, and the amount of themes that have been covered:

> 'Time flies when we get going about the old days; whatever we start talking about doesn't matter, we end up remembering so many different things.'

Roles played in groups

Important elements of groupwork knowledge are an understanding of the roles played by individuals in groups, and an awareness of the skills needed by the leader(s) to enhance the positive aspects of some roles and lessen the negative effects of others. The major influence of roles played by individuals in group processes is highlighted by Forsyth (1990):

> Roles in groups structure behaviour by dictating the 'part' that members take as they interact.

Valuable insights are gained into individuals' past behaviour in relation to others, and present attitudes towards group living, by observing and understanding the roles group members adopt in reminiscence sessions. The roles assumed by older people in groups may be exaggerated or altered by the force of dementia. Nevertheless, having an understanding of the basic roles individuals play in groups helps the leader(s) to interpret and handle the group process more sensitively. A group that consists of members playing different roles has a varied, colourful and lively atmosphere.

Examples of roles played in reminiscence groups include:

- *Information givers*, who enjoy recalling memories so that others will understand how life was in the past.
- *Advisors*, who like to be asked for their advice about how something would have been done in the past. They enjoy feeling knowledgeable about the past and competent in the present.
- *Observers*, who are often uncommunicative even when comments or questions are put to them directly; but who gain enjoyment from listening to and watching others. They may enjoy doing 'support' tasks for the group. For example, helping to tidy or wash up.
- *Recall 'experts'*, who experience very easy recall of memories. They enjoy the process greatly, bring energy to the group and are very stimulating in helping

to trigger memories in others. However, difficulties can arise with this role if the individual finds it hard to let others in, through a need to dominate the group process.

- *Supporters*, who are individuals good at connecting with others, and able to promote the group process by encouraging quieter members to participate.

THINKING POINT

Look back for a few minutes on any groups you have run. Can you think of individuals who adopted any of the above roles? How did you handle individuals who dominated the group process?

This is not an exhaustive list of roles played in reminiscence or other kinds of groups. Also, group members may move between roles, depending on factors such as their mood and physical health; the attitude of other members, and the style of group leadership. Often, but not always, one role is dominant for each individual. It is this dominant role that provides the greatest insights.

Suggestions on how to deal with difficulties that arise in the group process due to roles adopted by individual members in reminiscence sessions is included in Chapter 4, 'Running and Maintaining Group Reminiscence'.

POSITIVE GAINS THROUGH GROUPWORK

The general advantages of working in a reminiscence way with older people were discussed in detail in Chapter 1. There are, however, specific benefits to be gained by older people from involvement in the group reminiscence process:

- Social interaction with peers provides entertainment, communication, and the opportunity to build a closer relationship with other residents and staff.

- Group identity grows, creating a feeling of belonging, acceptance and purpose.

- Memories are stimulated by the collective discussion of common themes, making recall more enjoyable for all.

- Group activities that have their roots in the past. For example, preparing traditional dishes, which provide the opportunity to take part in 'doing' tasks, which are particularly effective in promoting recall. Within these group activities, taking an active part in the preparation process stimulates memories.

- Shared experiences around loss through bereavement, disability or dependence, reduce feelings of isolation and normalise older people's experience of grief.

Summary Points

Promoting Reminiscence

- Possessing underlying key attitudes, which acknowledge the value and uniqueness of older people and their histories is fundamental to the promotion of sensitive reminiscence work.
- Willingness on the part of carers to develop skills and knowledge in the areas of communication and groupwork enhances the reminiscence experience for older people.
- To listen and respond effectively carers need to 'tune in' to both verbal and non-verbal messages.
- Carers need to be able to hear and respond to the expression of strong feelings about past and present events.
- The process of group reminiscence can provide many benefits for older people, in part due to the sharing of the many common threads that run through the life experience of individuals.

3 Reminiscence Groups – *The Planning Stage*

It's funny how our memories group is only a bit of something but it really perks me up.
IRENE

TAKING THE INITIATIVE FOR PLANNING

Who is introducing group reminiscence in your work setting? The idea may have been suggested by a unit manager, with the aim of enhancing the programme of available weekly activities. An activity worker may be looking to revise an existing range of activities within a care setting, or to develop current reminiscence practice. Alternatively, carers within dementia units in homes or day-care settings may be looking to develop a daily programme of reminiscence-based activities.

Whatever the role and aim of carers planning to initiate reminiscence groupwork, the support of management and other colleagues will be essential. Inevitably, not all staff view reminiscence work as worthwhile or skilled; many view the activity as an 'easy option'. Discouraging and negative attitudes about the value of reminiscence work expressed by staff directly or indirectly need to be challenged. To counter any negativity towards reminiscence work management needs to promote and support the activity unequivocally, emphasising the role it has to play in the social and emotional care of older people.

General staff meetings offer an ideal forum for introducing and discussing plans for a reminiscence programme. Staff not directly involved in the reminiscence activity can be helped through training to raise their awareness of the issues and benefits involved in the work. Short in-house sessions using a selection of the activities provided in this handbook would help to challenge negative views of reminiscence work. Additionally, all staff can be encouraged to play a role in supporting reminiscence work by contributing artefacts for use as triggers in the work; reminding and escorting individuals to the group venue; as 'guests' invited by the group to an old-fashioned tea party or cake-tasting; or sharing in the enjoyment of any displays that celebrate a group's achievement.

Feedback to staff not directly involved in the progress of the group week by week, or at the end of a block of sessions, is invaluable in promoting reminiscence work. Regular feedback also provides an opportunity to discuss any difficulties or advantages observed in residents attending the group.

The role of management

Managers of residential, hospital or day-care settings have the opportunity and responsibility to influence the standards of care provided by their staff group. Older people thrive emotionally, socially and physically in caring regimes that have a commitment to maintaining the uniqueness of individuals within institutional environments. Programmes of care that facilitate a warm, respectful atmosphere, with an emphasis on social contact, stimulation and meaningful activities, maintain and enhance self-esteem.

Kitwood and Bredin (1997) emphasize the value of maintaining the uniqueness of individuals. They describe regimes that pursue the preservation of individuality as conferring on older people 'the privilege of personhood'. To maintain personhood, Kitwood and Bredin firmly believe in the need to create a caring regime where there is a marriage between empathy for and personal knowledge of individuals.

Reminiscence group and one-to-one work provides the arena for increasing both empathy for and personal knowledge about older people. As a result, reminiscence work can play a major role in maintaining personhood through the illumination of older people's individuality.

For managers to successfully promote reminiscence work there are resource issues in terms of staffing, supervision, time and finance to be considered. In terms of groupwork these include:

- Identifying committed group leaders
- Allocating time for leaders' supervision with, wherever possible, an experienced reminiscence worker
- Arranging work rotas so that leaders are available for the lifetime of the group
- Building in time for leaders to prepare and debrief on each session.
- Ensuring, as far as possible, that conflicting demands are not made on the leaders' session times
- Allocating funds and time for the collection of reminiscence artefacts
- Planning feedback sessions for the staff group on how the sessions have progressed

The task of group leaders

The following is a checklist of the points to consider when planning a reminiscence group:

- How many group leaders will there be?

- What is the purpose of the group?
- How many group members will be included?
- Making the choice between an open or closed group.
- What will be the duration of each session, and how many sessions will there be in total?
- Identification of an appropriate venue.
- Mix of group members.
- Invitations.
- Issues about confidentiality.
- Session planning.
- Recording group content.
- Evaluation of group.

Sole leadership

Reminiscence groups run by only one leader have disadvantages for both group members and the worker. Without a co-worker, some situations in sessions become difficult or impossible to handle successfully. Take a typical scenario in a group where one or more group members need accompanying to the toilet by the group leader entailing what may be a lengthy absence. This event may happen a number of times, even during a short session. If there is only one leader, the session loses continuity; attention of the group will be lost and will have to be regained on each return; group members may leave the room during the leader's absence and have to be encouraged to return resulting in further disruption to the group process.

Sole leadership is problematic in situations where group members become upset about the content of the session or unrelated issues; the leader may have insufficient time to offer comfort without disrupting the flow of the group. Other disadvantages of sole leadership include being unable to give sufficient attention to quiet members to ensure they have the opportunity to take part in the group process. Also, if group members have sight or hearing difficulties, one leader may be unable to promote full individual involvement in the session. Hearing clearly in a group situation is very difficult for older people with even a minor hearing loss, and leaders will often be involved in repeating group members' comments individually, to ensure everyone keeps up with the flow of conversation. Individual support from the group leader is also necessary where individuals have sight difficulties; detailed description of visual triggers may be necessary, together with encouragement to feel the artefact if appropriate.

These are just a few examples of situations that are impossible or very difficult for one leader to handle and maintain group continuity. In addition, carefully planned reminiscence activities, which would flourish with co-leaders, may fail due to the pressure on one leader to simultaneously facilitate group activities and meet individual conflicting demands.

THINKING POINT

Have you run a group alone, either reminiscence-based or covering another activity? Do you feel that sole-leadership proved disadvantageous to the group?

Co-leadership

When thinking about the choice of group leaders there are advantages in considering various combinations. For example, workers who together offer a blend of reminiscence work experience and existing knowledge of the group could be one pairing; other co-leaders could include combinations of care worker and manager; activities worker and care worker; care worker and volunteer; visiting reminiscence worker and care worker.

A combination of group leaders that includes one worker with past experience of running reminiscence groups can be particularly valuable in transferring skills and helping the confidence of the less experienced worker. However, key issues in the effective pairing of co-leaders centre on their willingness to cooperate, avoid competition and make a commitment to sharing tasks, and agreement on common goals for the group. Essentially, co-leaders should like, trust and respect each other, while holding similar views about the value and role of reminiscence work.

Co-leaders will benefit from taking sufficient time to plan and prepare for both the initial setting up of groups and individual sessions. It is also important to allow time at the end of each session to discuss the process of the group, including observations about individual reactions to the content and to each other. As each session is reviewed group leaders build on their experience, learning all the time about what activities, styles of co-leadership and group composition work well and those that are less successful. It may be tempting, with pressure from other caring commitments, to curtail planning and reviewing time. However, leading reminiscence groups is a skilled process that takes time to prepare for and evaluate. The reminiscence process, group members and leaders are devalued by inadequate time and importance being allocated to the work.

Purpose of the group

One of the tasks of the co-leaders is to decide what purpose(s) they see the group fulfilling. The following is an outline of the main purposes of reminiscence groups:

1 To provide a recreational activity that is both informal and structured, which group members find socially stimulating and entertaining.

2 To increase emotional and social wellbeing by acknowledging and retaining individual uniqueness and promoting relationships with peers and staff.

3 To gain increased background knowledge about group members, to help greater personalisation of social and physical care patterns.

4 To provide a daily reminiscence-based programme of activities that has an emphasis on carers 'being with' rather than 'doing to' individuals.

When identifying the purpose(s) of reminiscence groups it is important to focus on the members to be included in the sessions and their specific individual and group needs. Leaders may feel several or all of the purposes outlined are applicable to group members' needs; alternatively, one purpose alone may stand out as particularly appropriate.

By considering the purpose of the group reminiscence process, group leaders are helped to increase their appreciation of the intricacy and value of the work, both to themselves and to older people. Clarity about what it is hoped group members and leaders will gain from the reminiscence process helps in the planning of individual sessions and in the final evaluation of the group.

THINKING POINT

Think of an older person who you feel would benefit from attending a reminiscence group. Do any of the purposes outlined meet their needs within the reminiscence process?

Number of group members

The optimum number of individuals in a group, run by two leaders, is between five and eight. Groups with a maximum of eight members enable leaders to provide individual attention when required. Older people with special needs, such as hearing or sight difficulties benefit from a small group situation. Equally, the greater the confusion of individuals, the smaller the group should be in order to promote an effective reminiscence experience (see also Chapter 5, 'Reminiscence Work and the Challenge of Dementia').

Choosing an open or closed group

Group leaders need to choose either an open or closed reminiscence group. An open group involves a membership that is not fixed in terms of numbers, and/or specific individuals. Usually, this type of group does not have an end date, and new individuals join all the time. As a result, there is a constant need to build group unity by establishing trust between existing and new members.

In establishments providing only temporary care, such as hospitals, acute mental health settings or respite units, where there is a continuously changing population of older people, an open reminiscence group may be the only workable option. The purpose of open groups does not necessarily differ from that of closed groups, but may be harder to achieve due to a regularly changing membership.

In a closed group, members are invited to join for the duration of the group sessions. At each session, the same individuals are encouraged to attend and if someone is absent no one takes their place. A closed group promotes continuity; security with the group process and other group members is more easily facilitated than in an open group, and leaders have time to increase their individual knowledge of group members. Each session of a closed group has the opportunity to pass through its successive phases of 'nurturing', 'energising', 'peaking' and 'relaxing'. In contrast, an open group is likely to remain focused longer on the 'nurturing' stage, with leaders having to spend a large proportion of each session introducing new individuals to other group members and the group process itself. As a result there is a limited period of time each session for moving into the developing phases of the group.

If the group is closed, all staff, including those not directly involved in the activity, are clear about who is attending, and the duration of the group. As a result, staff are able to remind group members about when the sessions take place.

Duration

An appropriate length for weekly groups is approximately 45–60 minutes, including time for refreshments. Groups run for people with dementia are more effective if they are shorter and more frequent (see Chapter 5, 'Reminiscence Work and the Challenge of Dementia').

Ideally, groups should meet on the same day and time each week. The timing of groups needs to take into account established routines around mealtimes, caring tasks or activities and any transport commitments. Group timings that incorporate morning coffee but end before lunch are usually popular. However, in many care settings the period after lunch may be a good time to run reminiscence sessions, if the only other available activity is an afternoon sleep. Six to eight sessions with a break before starting a new group allows time for evaluation and planning for future sessions.

Venue

It is important to consider carefully the choice of venue for group reminiscence sessions. Often, sessions are run in group members' own lounge, unit or ward, where there is a familiarity with the physical environment. Familiarity with a well-known environment can increase the sense of security felt by individuals, particularly members with sensory, mobility or mental health difficulties.

The disadvantages of not using an alternative venue to the group members' normal living space include difficulty in establishing clear start and finish times, with the normal activities of the room going on around the group. Also, members do not have a change of scene from their normal surroundings. Choosing a venue with a view of a garden or the local neighbourhood provides an added interest for the group. Using a staff room as a group venue can result in resentment, even if the room is not in regular use.

It is beneficial if the venue is the same for each group session. The room needs to be warm, with good ventilation and comfortable seating. Easy access for wheelchairs may be required and proximity to toilet facilities is important. If possible, facilities for making refreshments should be available in the room.

A major factor associated with choosing a venue is who will accompany members to the group. If individuals are coming to the venue from different units, it will be a demanding and time-consuming task for leaders to be solely responsible for accompanying group members. It is helpful if leaders are able to engage the support of unit staff in accompanying group members to the venue. Group timings need to allow for the time required in escorting group members to and from the venue. Where possible, one leader needs to be present at the venue, to provide a welcome as members gather, prior to the start of the group.

Who to invite

Leaders, with other staff members, need to consider who it would be appropriate to invite to attend the reminiscence group. One influencing factor in this choice is whether the group is planned for individuals from one or more units within the residential or day setting. Alternatively, group composition may consist of individuals who share common experiences, such as having lived or worked in the same neighbourhood.

Another factor to consider when identifying potential group members is the appropriateness of a group membership consisting of older people who are and are not experiencing dementia. This mix can be successful if the group is small, relationships between all the group members are generally good, and those included with dementia, although experiencing varying degrees of memory loss, retain pleasure in the recall of past memories. However, if it is felt that group members who are not experiencing dementia are likely to be critical of, or overly frustrated with, members who have dementia, it would be beneficial to run separate groups.

Try to avoid inviting individuals to the group who openly dislike each other; disagreements between individuals during group sessions may occur, and have to be handled at the time. However, including members from the outset who are hostile to one another creates unease within the group during the early, tentative stages of formation.

Invitations

Once the leaders of the group have decided who to invite to the group, it will be necessary to consider how to make the approach to prospective group members. It is valuable if leaders meet individually with potential group members, to explain about the group and to offer a personal invitation to join.

Before initiating a first meeting with a prospective group member, find out any background information that is available on file and from key workers. It is important to establish if there are sensitive issues arising from an individual's past or present situation; individuals may wish to talk about recent bereavements or admission to care, and such traumatic events may also influence how the idea of reminiscence is received. Gathering this kind of background information adds to the sensitivity and individuality of the leader's initial approach to potential group members. It may be beneficial, when leaders are not well known to potential group members, for the key worker or another trusted member of staff to accompany the group leader. Individuals may be more receptive to joining the group if a trusted carer feels the experience would be helpful to them.

Everyone has their own style of communication, but it is important to think beforehand about a form of words that describe clearly what a reminiscence group is, and what individuals hopefully gain from attending. The following is a suggestion on how to phrase an invitation:

> 'We are planning to run a memories group where you would have the chance to share your memories about the past and listen to the memories of others. We hope the group will be enjoyable and interesting to members. It will give you an opportunity to both remember the past and get to know other residents better.'

This initial meeting between group leader and potential group member begins the process of building a trusting relationship. Additionally, if the leader is able to allow sufficient time for the meeting, valuable background information can be obtained about the individual's past. Obtaining information about an individual's life helps leaders make an appropriate selection of relevant themes and triggers for group sessions. Furthermore, knowledge of background history promotes understanding of, and sensitivity to, comments made by individuals in reminiscence sessions.

One piece of information that it is important to be clear about from this initial meeting is how the individual wishes to be referred to in the group. An individual's name is a large part of their personal identity. When even a slightly deviated form to someone's correct name is used, it can be unsettling and confusing, particularly if the older person is new to a care setting. Individuals may always have been known by their second name or a nickname. Group leaders need to be sure individuals are referred to in the way they are most familiar and happy with as illustrated by this case study:

> A resident in a home was called Lucy by her family; staff took their cue from the relatives when talking to her. One day when she was annoyed with a member of staff, she retorted when called Lucy:
>
> 'Will you please stop calling me that. It's my middle name and only my daughter and son use it. I prefer to be called by my first name, Barbara, by people outside the family.'

An older person may like being called by a certain name by family or friends, but may object to others adopting the same form of address.

THINKING POINT

Have you ever called someone you are caring for by an incorrect name? What was their response? How did you feel when you realised your error?

Background information gathered about individuals is valuable as an initial tool for personalising the reminiscence process, and can be added to during the life of the group. Personal information helps group leaders to increase their awareness of the individuality of group members. Recording information gained from this initial meeting is useful for future reference (see the Group Member's Profile Form at the end of this chapter).

A written invitation, in addition to a verbal one, with full details of group timings and venue, values the individual and the activity. It also provides a prompt, helping individuals to keep the group in mind prior to the start and between sessions. Try to remember to inform relatives too: most will be interested, and some may be in a position to lend or donate triggers for use with the group.

Confidentiality

It is important that group leaders have discussed together what form recording of the group process will take. Additionally, there needs to be agreement about when it would be appropriate to share information about the group with other staff. For example, sharing information about group members and the group process usually takes place during supervision, which may include an evaluation of the group. However, it may also be beneficial to share information about specific group members, outside supervision, with care staff in order to facilitate an individual's care.

Most individuals know and accept that information is recorded about them, and will recall having to discuss their personal circumstances prior to being admitted to the residential, nursing or day setting. However, at the initial meeting with potential group members it is helpful to explain that additional background information is very useful when planning and running reminiscence sessions.

At the initial meeting of the group, it is important to remind group members about the issue of confidentiality, pointing out that it is helpful in building trust if everyone is confident that information shared in the sessions is not discussed outside the group. The only exception to this would be in instances where sharing information outside the group, with relevant members of staff, would be valuable in improving an individual's care. Reminders about the importance of group confidentiality may be necessary if, on occasion, individuals share information that is particularly personal or upsetting to them.

PLANNING SESSIONS – THE ROLE OF THEMES AND TRIGGERS

An effective way of running reminiscence groups is to base individual sessions on a theme. This provides the group with an initial focus of memory in each session. Themes can cover all aspects of life in the past; in addition, many themes have a role, albeit a changed one, in the lives of older people in the present. Generally contrasts between the past and today make for interesting and lively group discussion.

Leaders, through their initial discussions with group members, will have gained detailed information about members' past lives. There may be strong common threads running through group members' lives, which indicate a choice of themes that would be of general interest. For example, these themes might be related to where individuals lived, or jobs they held. In the absence of strong past links between group members, broad reminiscence themes based on general aspects of individuals' past lives will also be effective in promoting recall.

Broad reminiscence themes can be broken down into sub-themes. For example, the broad theme of 'Home' has the following sub-themes: neighbourhood; type of housing; neighbours; shopping; transport and traffic in street; walk to school; playing outside; housework; mealtimes; family rules. The list is far from exhaustive, and 'Home' is just one broad theme out of many. A list of appropriate themes and sub-themes effective in prompting memories in reminiscence groupwork are given in Chapter 4, 'Running and Maintaining Group Reminiscence'.

Triggers in reminiscence sessions are used to evoke memories by representing themes and sub-themes. Triggers include objects, photographs, music, poetry, sayings, smells, and flowers. The use of a variety of triggers that appeal to individuals' different senses of hearing, sight, touch, smell and taste are the most evocative in prompting memories. For example, if 'Home' is chosen as the theme of a session, and the sub-theme is 'Cleaning', the triggers used could include those listed in Table 6.

Table 6 · **SUB-THEME OF CLEANING – TRIGGERS AND SENSE APPEAL**

Triggers	Sense appeal
Objects:	
Scrubbing brush	Touch, sight
Carbolic soap	Sight, smell, touch
Red step polish	Sight, smell
Photographs:	
Old adverts for cleaning materials and Hoovers	Sight
Quotes	
'It was my job, as the oldest girl in the family to blacklead the grate every Friday.'	Hearing
'My mother polished our front step with cardinal red polish every week, as did all our neighbours.'	

Reminiscence groups focusing on the theme of 'Cleaning' may not need all the listed triggers to prompt memories; one trigger only may be sufficient to stimulate a chain of memories. It is important not to overwhelm individuals with too many stimuli; often, two or three objects placed on a table in the middle of the group will be sufficient to prompt recall of memories. Additional triggers can be kept in reserve to use, if needed, later in a session. Once a group member shares a recollection, others, in turn, are stimulated to recall memories associated or disconnected with the initial memory.

Triggers that engage group members in a 'doing' process, such as helping to prepare traditional foods, or polishing brasses, are usually particularly successful in prompting recall of memories. Familiar actions from the past, coupled with the stimulus of appropriate triggers, stir memories in the present.

Planned themed sessions are important in promoting positive reminiscence work. However, it is essential that group leaders are able to let the group take control in choosing the emphasis of recall, even if this is off at a tangent from the original theme. Group members often share memories that diverge from the session's planned theme, provoking in some group leaders a sense of failure:

> 'The group had wanted to talk about schooldays as our planned theme for the session, and I had taken along triggers including old school inkwells, photographs of old local school buildings and children at a school fete. I only had a chance to show the group the photograph of the school fete before they were quickly diverging from the theme, talking about the jobs they had when they left school. We did not return, in that session, to the theme of school. I felt the group was out of my control, and that I was not a good leader unless I could bring them back to talk about what we had agreed.'

The success of reminiscence groups is not derived from group leaders' control over recall of specific areas of memory, but from the enjoyment, stimulation and sociability experienced by group members from taking part in the process of reminiscing. Individuals illustrate their enjoyment and spontaneity within the group reminiscence process when they have the interest and confidence to diverge from planned themes.

Trigger collection

A collection of triggers is invaluable in promoting group reminiscence work. To start a collection, engage the help of other staff, relatives and friends to lend or donate any items that may be of interest. In the same way that themes can be as varied as life itself, so can the kinds and sources of triggers. For example, think about objects in everyday use today in the home: was there an equivalent in the past that older people would remember?

Good sources for triggers are charity shops, car boot and jumble sales. In addition, local organisations working with older people, for example Age Concern (in Britain), have collections of artefacts. Many libraries and heritage museums also have themed boxes for hire, which contain objects and photographs on many areas of local life in the past.

The initial session

In the first session with members new to the reminiscence process, and possibly to other group members, it is helpful for leaders to have a clear plan about an appropriate theme for the session. It is important to encourage all group members to take part in the initial session, to help individuals feel at ease with each other, the leaders, and the process of reminiscence itself. Choosing a broad theme such as 'Home', 'Schooldays' or 'Work', that is likely to be of common interest to group members, promotes the greatest involvement of members.

In subsequent sessions it is important to encourage 'ownership' of the group by its members, which can be achieved in part through encouraging the group to choose the themes for discussion each week. Initially, members may say they do not mind what is discussed; however, if leaders offer some ideas for themes, preferences are often stated.

RECORDING GROUP SESSIONS

To enhance group leaders' work in the reminiscence field, evaluation of sessions is vital, both for new and established group leaders.

Following each group session, leaders should ideally have an opportunity for sharing impressions about the session. Difficulties and positive aspects of the session should be discussed, and plans made for the next session. The Weekly Reminiscence Group Review Form included at the end of this chapter has been designed for use in recording session content.

EVALUATION

At the finish of the group, the weekly review forms could form part of the overall evaluation of the group, together with a consideration of whether the purpose(s) identified at the planning stage of the group have been achieved. It is helpful if this evaluation is carried out with a supervisor experienced in reminiscence work. Groupwork evaluation offers an opportunity to look at the achievements of the group, and to determine what changes are needed to add to the value of future groups. Group evaluations are often the appropriate point to draw together knowledge about individuals acquired through the group process. This information can be used to enhance future patterns of care.

Reminiscence groupwork is a skilled process, with demands on staff time and other resources. The preparation process outlined in this chapter is detailed, and it may be tempting to allow insufficient time for each stage of planning and evaluation. However, staff enjoyment and expertise in reminiscence work will be enhanced if sufficient time is provided for preparing, running and evaluating group sessions. Older people, in turn, will quickly come to value the opportunity to be part of a structured, well-planned and purposeful activity. Figure 2 summarises the stages in planning a reminiscence group.

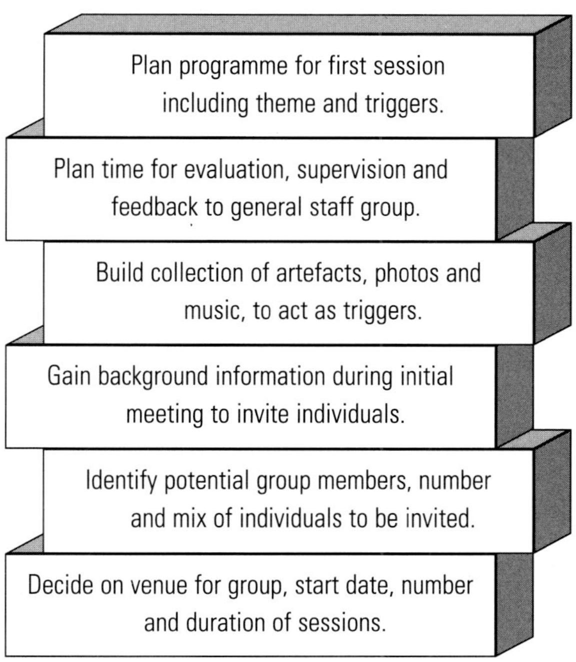

Figure 2 Building blocks in planning a reminiscence group

Summary Points

Reminiscence Groups – Planning

- Leaders of reminiscence groups need the support of other colleagues when introducing or developing this activity.
- Reminiscence groupwork contributes to the creation of climates of care in establishments that foster the maintenance and celebration of individuals' uniqueness.
- Positive reminiscence work requires a commitment of staff time, and supervisory and financial resources.
- Joint rather than sole leadership is most effective in promoting a positive reminiscence process.
- Planning, prior to setting up and during the life of reminiscence groups, and evaluation following completion, contribute to the success of the activity.

Group Member's Profile Form

Name of group member ______________________ Date of birth ____________

Date of admission ______________________________________

Sources of information **1** Staff ☐ **2** Files ☐ **3** Group Member ☐ **4** Relatives/friends ☐

Former home address ______________________________________

____

____

____

How individual prefers to be addressed ______________________________________

____

Marital status ______________________________________

Partner's name ______________________________________ Deceased ☐ Y/N

Partner's occupation ______________________________________

Children's names ______________________________________

____

Areas where children live ______________________________________

Grandchildren's names ______________________________________

____

Other close friends/relatives eg, siblings ______________________________________

____

____

Area lived in as a child, if known ______________________________________

Parents' names ______________________________________

Parents' occupations ______________________________________

Group Member's Profile Form *continued*

Own occupation(s) and/or voluntary work ______________________

____

____

____

Hobbies, interests and skills ______________________

____

____

____

Places and events of special importance ______________________

____

____

Reasons for their importance ______________________

What member is proud to have achieved ______________________

____

____

Themes that may have particular interest or significance ______________________

____

____

____

Other significant information ______________________

____

____

____

____

____

Form completed by ______________________ *Date* ______________

Weekly Reminiscence Group Review Form

Session number ______________________________ Date ____________________

Who attended ____

____

Planned theme ____

Triggers used ____

Group process

Response to theme and triggers used ________________________________

____

Was the theme of general interest to group? __________________________

____

Were all triggers used to promote recall of memories? __________________

Which trigger(s) were most successful in promoting recall of memories? ________

____

Which senses were particularly stimulated by the triggers used? ___________

____

Examples of comments made by group members, using their own words as far as possible

____

____

____

____

Group members' response to each other and the leader(s) _______________

____

____

____

Was the atmosphere one of general sharing and enjoyment in remembering? ______

____

Weekly Reminiscence Group Review Form
continued

Were any negative comments made between members? How were these handled by group leader(s)?

Was the group dominated by one or two very talkative members?

How did group leader(s) handle this or other difficult situations in the group?

Ideas and strategies for coping with any difficult group interactions in future sessions

Overall view of session

Additional information gained about individual group members that could be used to enhance their care

Suggested theme and associated triggers for next session

4 Running and Maintaining Group Reminiscence

I would tell you the tale of my life, sir, but I don't want my tea to get cold.
JOHN KILLICK, *Monkey Puzzle, Please Give Me Back My Personality! Writing and Dementia*

GETTING STARTED

Having completed the preparatory work involved in setting up a reminiscence group as detailed in Chapter 3 the format of the first session needs to be planned.

Taking part in, or setting up, something new can be daunting and it is possible both group leaders and members may feel a mixture of concern and anticipation about how the group sessions will work out. Group members may know each other individually as fellow residents, day users or patients, but being together for a group activity may be a new experience.

Group members, although having initially agreed to take part in the reminiscence activity, may at the last minute feel they prefer the known and secure pattern of their days to this new experience. Alternatively, individuals may be familiar with informal reminiscing on a one-to-one basis with carers, but be less sure about how the process works or feels in a structured group situation. Group leaders may find, immediately prior to the start of the first session, that time is needed to remind group members about the format of the group, and what it is hoped will be gained from the experience.

Gathering together

To ease any apprehension on the part of group members, it is important that as individuals gather they are greeted by one of the leaders and helped to find a seat, if possible next to a known and liked fellow member.

Once everyone has arrived, leaders should offer a general welcome. It is helpful at this beginning stage to reiterate what a memories group is, and what it is hoped group members will gain from the experience of attending the group. Individuals may be concerned about how long they will be away from their familiar surroundings and routines; it is important to provide information about how long the session will last each week, and the number of weeks the group will run.

Reassurance can be offered about group members being escorted back to their lounge at the end of the meeting. Some individuals may be concerned about missing their morning or afternoon drinks, or finding the toilet in new surroundings. Practical concerns such as these can be anticipated and reassurances offered. Take these initial explanations slowly, giving group members time to settle and feel more at ease with the new surroundings and each other.

THINKING POINT

Reflect on a recent occasion when you attended a training session through work, or a personal situation when you were in a group where some or all of the other members were strangers. How did the group leader encourage introductions? How did you feel in this situation? Do you enjoy meeting new people in group settings? Or do you try to avoid these situations?

Breaking the ice

A warm welcome and introductions by group leaders help to create a secure and sociable atmosphere in an initial group session. An icebreaker activity at the beginning of the session promotes enjoyable contact between group members. The most appropriate icebreakers are those that provide the opportunity for all group members to join in the process of getting to know other members during the initial phase of group formation. Learning names at the start of any group can be difficult; one icebreaker that helps this process involves encouraging group members to throw a soft foam ball (some are available that make a noise when caught) around the group circle. When a member catches the ball, they are asked to tell the group their name. Usually this icebreaker helps to ease initial tensions in groups, providing an enjoyable activity while helping members to get to know each other.

As members relax and start to enjoy themselves, group leaders can introduce the memories theme for the session. In this first session it will have been necessary for the group leaders to identify a theme. In subsequent sessions, group members with a developing sense of ownership of the group should be encouraged to suggest themes.

Choice of themes

It is helpful in this initial session to choose a theme (see Chapter 3, 'Reminiscence Groups – The Planning Stage', and later in this chapter for a list of possible themes and triggers) that is likely to have general interest for group members, but is not associated with painful memories. It may be difficult and upsetting if, in the first session, there is a heavy emotional content to memories shared. But it is obviously not possible to guarantee that any theme, however seemingly innocuous, will not hold the power to evoke painful memories for some individuals. Additionally, for everyone, the past holds positive and more difficult memories, and no one is able to choose to recall only the good times. During the lifetime of any group, leaders and group members are likely to have to respond to painful memories expressed by individuals. However, the expression and acceptance of emotions will be easier as individuals get to know and trust group leaders and each other.

In introducing the theme of a session, it is helpful to put the related triggers on a low table in the middle of the group. Just seeing a certain trigger may stimulate recollections of the past, resulting in one or more group members recalling their memories. Alternatively, one of the leaders could hold up one of the triggers and ask the group generally if the object is familiar to them, or if anyone had a similar object. Be patient: do not rush on with several questions; let the group take its time. As individuals begin sharing their memories, be aware of the need to try to involve everyone in the group to avoid individuals feeling left out, particularly during this early stage in the group process. However, remember that group members can be involved, without necessarily contributing verbally, by enjoying listening to others or just looking at the triggers. Group leaders can facilitate involvement by moving around the group circle, making sure everyone has the chance to see and hold the triggers.

As group members recollect and share memories triggered by the session's theme they attain pleasure and stimulation from remembering the past. In this first session, as in subsequent sessions, content of memories is less important than individual enjoyment in the process of recall and the growth of group cohesion that develops from a sense of togetherness in remembering.

Drawing up ground rules

One of the tasks of group leaders is to ensure that all group members have a positive reminiscence experience. A key element in achieving this task is to promote respect between all individuals in the group. Ground rules make an important contribution to creating an atmosphere of trust and mutual respect in reminiscence groupwork sessions. In any group situation where personal memories are shared, it is essential that all individuals receive good attention, respect and understanding.

It is difficult for group leaders to try to draw up ground rules about how individuals should be with each other at the start of the initial session; at this point, group members may find it difficult to understand what is being asked of them. However, if the idea of ground rules is broached towards the end of the session, leaders may be able to give concrete examples from the group process that illustrate the need to look at how the reminiscence experience can be improved for all group members.

If, for example, one of the issues in the session has been group members talking over each other, the leaders could illustrate how this caused difficulties:

> 'Everyone had lots of memories about using a dolly for washing, and suddenly you were all talking at once and we missed hearing so many memories. Perhaps one thing we could agree is to try to talk one at a time. It won't always work, but if you agree we could remind you when everyone is talking at once. What do you think?'

Emphasising the need as part of the agreement to respect different views and ways of living may be illustrated by reminding the group that:

> 'From the memories already shared it shows the varied lives you have all lived. It is important that we all value and respect different backgrounds and beliefs. Do you agree?'

Helping group members to understand that recalling memories can be painful as well as pleasurable is important if individuals are to accept the expression of emotion by themselves and others in sessions. The group can be helped to acknowledge this by explaining that:

> 'The memories group is aimed at giving you enjoyment in the recall of memories, but it is important to realise that remembering may be painful. It often helps to cry or express other emotions about sad times, and if we can understand and accept someone's pain they will not feel embarrassed but helped by the group. Is that something you would agree with?'

Gaining agreement about the importance of confidentiality is another area to discuss with group members:

> 'We hope that as we spend time together in the group trust between us will grow. One way to achieve this is to feel sure that what is shared in sessions will not be discussed outside the group. As group leaders, we also need to respect confidentiality. But we would like your general permission to share information disclosed in the group with other staff when it relates directly to the present care of individuals. Does this sound all right to you all?'

Gaining agreement about a set of ground rules in the early stages of the group process provides a sensitive framework within which group members can relate to each other. Additionally, if difficulties arise in the group process, individuals can be reminded about the group's ground rules.

THINKING POINT

Have you, as the leader or member of a group been involved in drawing up ground rules? How successful were these ground rules in creating a positive group process?

Refreshments

Providing refreshments is a valuable way of creating an enjoyable and relaxing atmosphere in a group. There is no right or wrong time to provide a refreshment break: if a morning start time for the session coincides with the group members' usual coffee time, it will be important to offer refreshments at the beginning of the group. In this instance, refreshments would signify a welcome to group members, and ensure the continuance of a familiar and secure routine.

Talking can be thirsty work, and refreshments at the end of the group are a pleasant and relaxing way of rounding off the session. Additionally, if a session is struggling to gain momentum, pausing to have a drink could help the group members to feel more at ease with each other, and encourage the memories to flow.

Endings

It is important to 'round off' the session by asking individuals if they enjoyed the group, sharing too what the leaders have enjoyed. Sum up by reminding the group what general memories have been shared, and asking group members for ideas for a theme for the following week (suggesting ideas to choose from if necessary). Finally, it is important to bring group members back to the here and now by reminding them that the group is finishing shortly, but will meet again next week.

PROMOTING THE FLOW OF FUTURE GROUP SESSIONS

With the introductory first session over, thoughts will turn to ideas for maintaining interest in the group and promoting a positive ongoing reminiscence experience. To achieve this, it is helpful to look at what general factors influence the success of reminiscence groups.

Content of sessions

One of the most important elements in promoting ongoing positive group reminiscence work is the use of themes and triggers that bring memories to life for older people (see also Chapter 3, 'Reminiscence Groups – The Planning Stage'). Effective themes in reminiscence work relate to broad areas of older people's past lives. Triggers are used to represent chosen themes and can cover a range of objects including equipment used in cleaning, washing, cooking, leisure or work activities; smells; music; photographs; flowers. To be effective triggers need to:

- Appeal to different senses, which is particularly important if group members have sensory loss in one or more areas.

- Be relevant to all cultures represented in the group.
- Be practical to handle.

Triggers have a varied role to play in stirring and illuminating memories for older people. Many enjoy looking at or holding objects from the past; for others, pleasure is gained from describing, and possibly miming, the past uses of objects. Listening to well-loved songs from the past is also often evocative as is the process of taking part in a familiar past activity, such as preparing traditional food, potting up bulbs, or planting seeds and cleaning brasses.

Seasonal triggers from nature, for example, garden or wild flowers, fruit, conkers and autumn leaves are effective in promoting recall. Smells associated with cake- or bread-making, cleaning materials, favourite perfumes, scents or flowers all have the power to transport individuals back to another time and place.

Where groups have a mixed cultural composition, it is important that triggers chosen to represent session themes have a relevance to all group members. Some older people may have emigrated many years before from their country of birth, so triggers relating, for example, to themes connected to childhood and young adulthood will need to be culturally-specific in order to facilitate recall (see also Chapter 6, 'Reminiscence Work across Cultures').

Triggers and sensory loss

If there are some group members with sensory loss in the areas of hearing or sight, it will be important to consider how their enjoyment of triggers can be maximised. Many older people have some degree of visual difficulty, and the use of a magnifying glass or magnification sheet may be sufficient to enhance enjoyment of photographs or pictures. Computer scanning and photocopying can also be used to enlarge photographs and pictures. Using slides both increases visibility and allows the group to view images simultaneously. However, the advantages of using slides have to be weighed against the disadvantages of working in a darkened room and losing the closeness of sitting in a circle. Additionally the noise of a projector can be frustrating for those group members with hearing loss. A recent innovation is the multimedia projector, which in the future will have an important role to play in improving the effectiveness of the use of photographs in reminiscence work.

Where group members have little or no residual sight, it will be essential to have available triggers that appeal to their remaining senses of touch, taste, smell and hearing. Older people with visual loss can also be encouraged to hold and touch triggers while the group leader describes the object.

Hearing loss in group members can make communication in groups a frustrating experience even for those wearing hearing aids. Difficulties can be minimised by working in small groups; leaders sitting near members with hearing loss and repeating other members' comments; using sufficient triggers that appeal to the surviving senses of touch, taste, smell and sight; and using aids that amplify sounds.

Rides into the country or to the seaside provide 'vistas' of natural triggers for older people with or without sensory loss. Many older people have lived in or visited the country or seaside during their past lives; the sight, sounds and smells of nature offer pleasure in the present and stimulus to recall the past.

> Vera's eyesight was slowly deteriorating. She could no longer read books or newspapers, and often became distressed about her lack of sight. The theme of one reminiscence group session Vera attended was a ride out to the local countryside where she had lived as a child. Vera became animated during the trip expressing pleasure at the sights around her. She spoke of the bold greens and yellows of spring, and a feeling of 'coming alive' again; she was in an environment which was large and full of loud colour, which her failing eyesight was still able to register. The largely unchanged natural environment helped her recall memories of long walks taken as a child.

As illustrated in Vera's case, in instances of severe sensory loss, triggers can be identified that enable individuals to participate enjoyably in reminiscence sessions.

When working with individuals with sensory loss it is important to ensure that there has been an up-to-date assessment of their needs, and that appropriate aids or equipment have been obtained. Specialist organisations exist at a local and national level in Britain, the USA and Australia, to provide advice on aids and equipment for people with visual and hearing difficulties.

GENERAL THEMES AND TRIGGERS

The themes and associated triggers suitable for use in reminiscence work are extensive. The following pages suggest a range of themes and triggers that could provide a 'starter pack' for group leaders. They include ideas for themes that involve a 'doing' element, which provide the opportunity for group members to take part in hands-on activities that would have been familiar in the past. Including a 'doing' element in session themes creates opportunities for evocative recall in the present.

The importance of obtaining a collection of triggers representing as many themes as possible cannot be over-emphasized. Such collections provide pleasure for older people both during the reminiscence process and, in a more general way, when collections are on permanent display. Objects from the past bring life and interest to reminiscence activities, helping to focus and facilitate the recall of memories.

THEMES WITH A 'DOING' ELEMENT

Eating and drinking

Trigger ideas Traditional recipe books, old weighing scales, crock pastry bowls, rolling pins, jam 'kettles'.

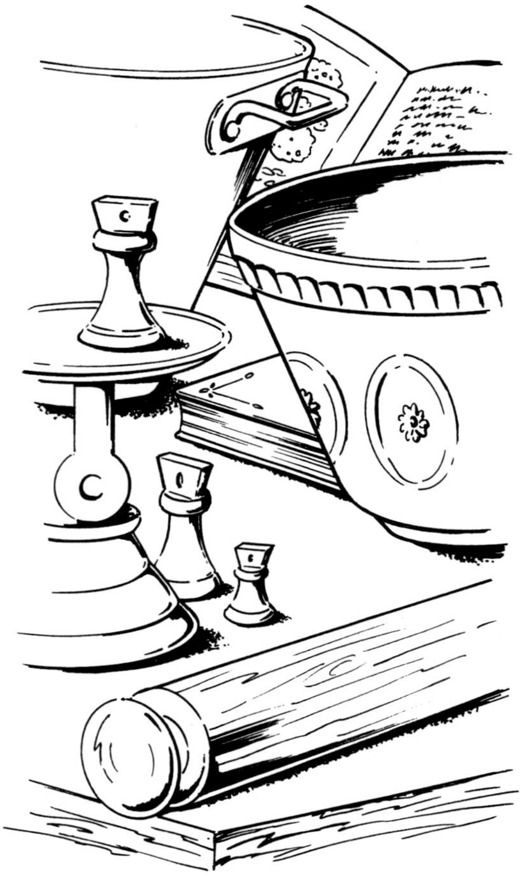

Hands-on activities Preparing and cooking food with group members taking a turn in mixing, weighing ingredients, rolling pastry or preparing cake tins.
Making home-made wine or jam using traditional ingredients: potato, dandelion, elderberry.
Making dumplings, cocoa bread and patties.

Note:

1 When preparing traditional food where there is a cultural mix of group members, all cultures need to be represented in the choice of traditional dishes.

2 Traditional food can also be prepared by groups to mark special celebrations. For example, Christmas and Easter, Thanksgiving and Independence Day.

Trigger ideas Crock teapots, leaf tea and tea strainer, traditional tea-set and tablecloth.

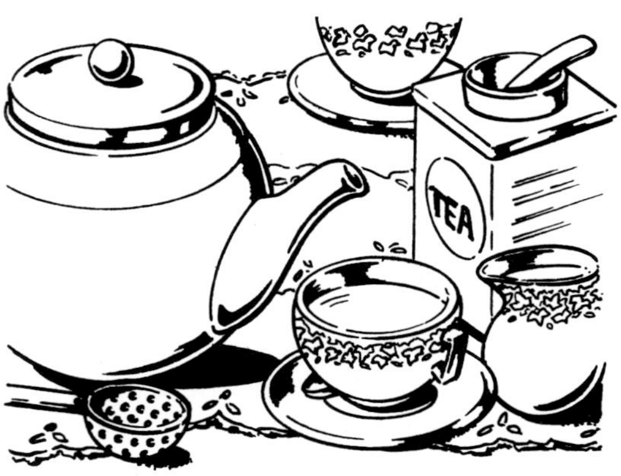

Hands-on activities
Advising/helping to make a traditional afternoon cup of tea.

Cleaning and washing

Trigger ideas Blue-bag, metal cleaner, starch, carbolic soap, scrubbing brush, floor polish, wooden washboard and dolly, quotes about washdays.

Hands-on activities Cleaning brasses/silver.
Starching.
Folding sheets.

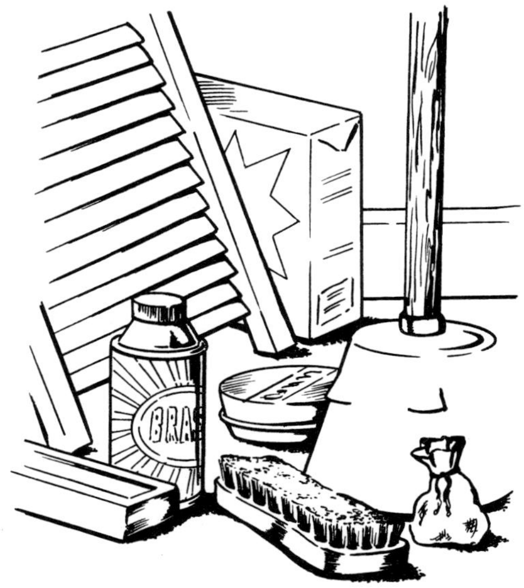

Sewing

Trigger ideas Treadle or wheel-operated sewing machine, button box, dress-making patterns, wooden mushroom for darning socks.

Hands-on activities Group members helped to use sewing machines and cut out dress patterns.
Rag-rugging.

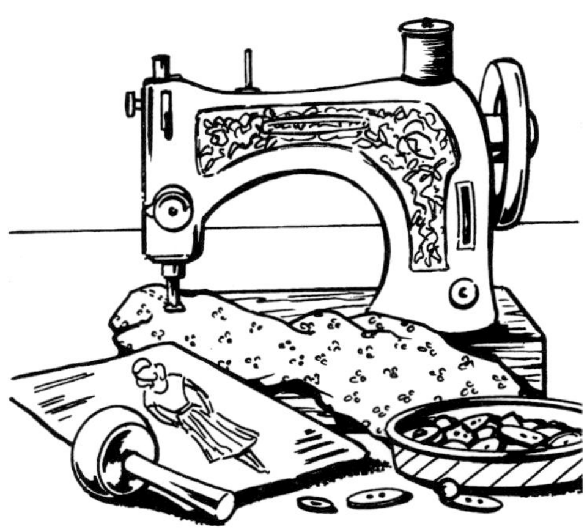

Clothes

Trigger ideas Hats, gloves, shoes, furs, evening bags, photographs showing examples of clothes from the 1920s to the 1950s.

Hands-on activities Trying on clothes from the past.
Smelling and applying perfume.

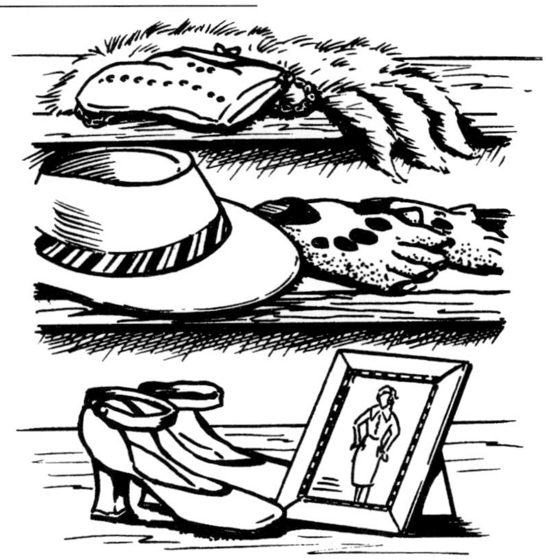

Music

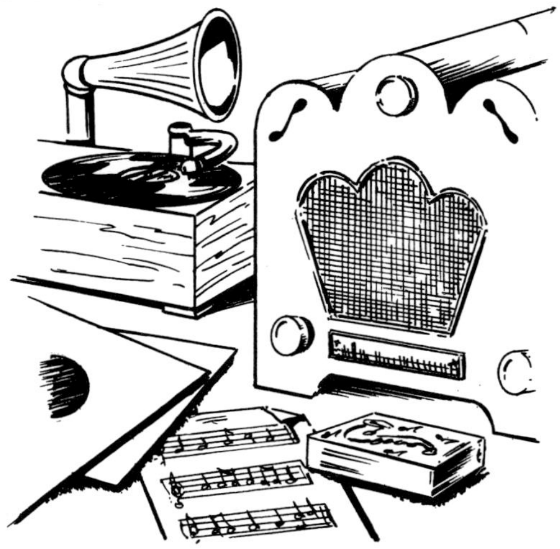

Trigger ideas Compilation tapes of music, song sheets, tape music quizzes – for example Speechmark *Sing Along* tape, *Sounds Nostalgic* tape of Famous Voices and Radio Themes from 1940s and 1950s, radios and gramophones from 1930 to 1960s.

Hands-on activities Singing, clapping and dancing to music.
Traditional dancing.

Outings

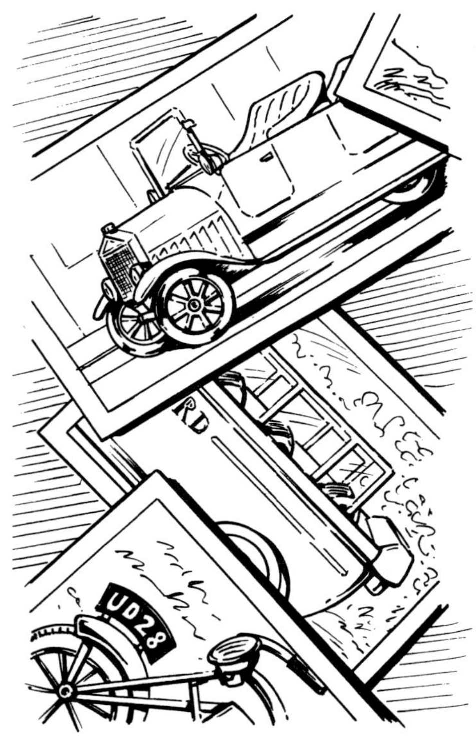

Trigger ideas Photographs of transport from the past: cars and motorbikes, charabancs from 1920 to 1950s. Quotes about days out at the seaside or in the country.

Hands-on activities Outings to local well-known beauty spots. Meals out at group members' 'local'.
Take-away with an old fashioned flavour, eg, fish and chips.
Visits to local industrial museums.

Gardening

Trigger ideas Old gardening books and equipment, seed packets, galvanised watering cans.

Hands-on activities Giving advice and overseeing planting and maintenance of vegetable plot. Helping plant and care for seeds and bulbs.

THINKING POINT

Can you think of an older person who would enjoy being practically involved in one of the 'doing' themes listed? Which one is it, and what would they enjoy about the experience?

THEMES: IDEAS FOR PROMPTING QUESTIONS AND TRIGGERS

Home life

***Prompting questions*:**

- What is your earliest memory of home?
- Where was your childhood home?
- What family routines and rules were there?
- What job did your parent(s) or carers do?
- What help did you have to give in the home?
- Did you have a favourite grandparent or uncle or aunt?
- What were mealtimes like in your home?
- Were there set days for washing and cleaning?

***Ideas for triggers*:**

- Photographs of group members' local neighbourhoods as they were in their childhood.
- Read out published quotes from older people about childhood in the past.
- Flat irons, washboards, washing dolly.
- Moth balls. Old lighting equipment: white-wax candles, storm lanterns and paraffin lamps.

Neighbourhood

***Prompting questions*:**

- What was your street like when you lived there as a child?
- If you lived in the country, were you in a village or on an isolated farm?
- Imagine standing at the back door, or on the front step of your childhood home: what would you have seen?
- Did tradesmen come up the street selling their goods?
- What did they sell?
- What views of the countryside could you see?
- Were there local shops, cinemas or dance halls?
- What were the neighbours like?
- Were you far from your parents/carers' work?
- What games did you play in the street or fields?
- Were you allowed out on your own?

***Ideas for triggers*:**

- Photographs of houses similar to those that group members' lived in. Artefacts associated with childhood games: conkers, skipping ropes, marbles.
- Draw a hopscotch outside, and ask group members to tell you how they played the game.
- Offer to draw the street where a group member lived, while they talk about it, including their own home and neighbours' houses, and other buildings in the street (only a basic drawing is required). This helps prompt an individual's memory, so they can visualise what they are describing.

Schooldays

***Prompting questions*:**

- How far away from home was your school?
- How did you get there? Did you have a favourite or particularly disliked teacher?
- What was your favourite subject at school?
- Did you have a 'nit nurse' visit your school?
- Did you have a best friend?
- Was anyone bullied at school?
- Did anyone get the cane?
- How old were you when you left school?
- Do you remember any smells from school, eg, carbolic soap, wet clothes, disinfectant?
- Let's try saying some of the times tables together.

***Ideas for triggers*:**

- Photographs of old schoolrooms.
- Read out short extracts from poems learned at school.
- Ink wells.
- Chalk.
- Slate boards.
- Carbolic soap.
- Jeyes fluid.
- School bell.

Work

***Prompting questions*:**

- What was your first job?
- About how much did you earn?
- What sort of things did you spend your wages on?
- Did you stay in the same job for a long time?
- As a woman did you have to give up your job when you got married or did you go on working?
- Did anyone take work into the home to do?
- What local industries were there to provide work when you left school?

- Did anyone leave the local area to find work?
- Did you have the chance to stay on at school to take qualifications?

***Ideas for triggers*:**
- Photographs or quotes about local industries in the area where individuals worked.
- In the UK, pre-decimal coins to represent the weekly wage paid.
- Artefacts used in individuals' workplaces.
- Visits to museums where exhibits about local industries are on display.

Setting up home

***Prompting questions*:**
- What were the traditions of courtship in those days?
- Did you live with in-laws?
- How did you furnish your home?

***Ideas for triggers*:**
- Quotes from relevant cultures about marriage traditions.
- Group members' photographs of their weddings.

Festivals and bank holidays

***Prompting questions*:**
- Which festivals or bank holidays did you celebrate?
- How were these celebrated?
- What did you wear?
- What beliefs and traditions were there around marriage, birth and death?
- Where did you go for days out?
- How did you get there?

***Ideas for triggers*:**
- Photographs of relevant traditional festivals.
- Photographs of public transport vehicles and popular seaside towns.

Dressing up

***Prompting questions*:**
- Do you remember your first outfit?
- How did you save up for special clothes?
- Where would you go for a night out?
- What was your favourite going out outfit?
- How much was a pair of stockings those days?
- What were the rules about the time you had to be in at night?
- What happened if you didn't make the deadline?

Ideas for triggers:
- In the UK, pre-decimal money.
- Stockings or fancy gloves.
- Make up.
- Hats.
- Evening bags.

Wartime

***Prompting questions*:**
- Can you remember any slogans from the war?
- How did you manage on small rations for clothes and food?
- What was the best and worst thing about the war?

***Ideas for triggers*:**
- Ration books.
- Reading out the weekly ration quota for food, and war slogans.
- Playing short extracts of famous speeches made by politicians or royalty, and well-known songs of the day.

POINTERS TO THINK ABOUT WHEN CHOOSING THEMES

Certain themes, for example weddings, having children, wartime, hold the potential for prompting emotionally laden recall for older people. For some individuals in a group memories of their wedding day may trigger painful thoughts and feelings about the death of a spouse. Alternatively, some men and women may not have married and feel resultant loss and regret about missing the experience. Similarly, when discussing childbirth, a proportion of women in a group may have experienced a stillbirth or miscarriage and still have unresolved feelings of loss about the event; others may not have had children and regret this. Issues about adoption also figure largely in a number of older people's lives. The war too is often an emotionally charged theme, many older people having experienced the untimely deaths of members of their family during wartime.

Reminiscence research prior to beginning memories work may alert leaders to areas of recall that could be painful for certain individuals. However, it is not possible to avoid all hurtful recall for older people and, if group leaders handle the expression of emotions sensitively, individuals may obtain some relief following the sharing of painful feelings. Additionally, the enjoyment in remembering a happy event, for instance a wedding, may provide consolation in coping with the ongoing sadness about the subsequent loss of a partner. Equally, recalling the comradeship experienced in wartime may help counter some of the feelings of loss about this traumatic period in an individual's life. Sensitivity to, and acknowledgement of, painful feelings also help to smooth the process of recall about uncomfortable memories.

ROLE OF PERSONAL POSSESSIONS

Many older people enjoy bringing photographs and other personal possessions to group sessions. Group members who do this show that they are enjoying the group process and are very open to sharing their past life with the group. However, sensitivity is needed on the part of the group leader in relation to the circumstances of the other group members: large numbers of older people move to care settings without the opportunity to choose what to bring with them and, as a result, lose cherished possessions.

When a group member attends a session with numerous personal possessions there is a possibility that the individual will dominate the group for a lengthy period. If this situation arises, it is important that the group leader avoids other group members feeling excluded. One way of avoiding this dominance of the group process is to thank the individual after they have recalled their initial memory about their possessions, stating that you are sure this recollection will have helped other group members recall their own memories. At this point the leader looks away in order to bring others into the group process.

THINKING POINT

Think for a moment about an older person you care for, or have cared for, who has shared with you their feelings about losing a cherished possession(s) as a result of moving to care. What was the object they lost and what feelings did they express when talking about the loss?

MAINTAINING GROUP COMMUNICATION

Ideas for icebreakers

At the beginning of group sessions, even when a group has previously met for several sessions, group members and leaders may feel uneasy, experiencing a sense of having to start again. Quickly establishing a sense of being together and trust is an important role for group leaders. Icebreakers are invaluable in reducing initial group tensions, providing enjoyable activities with the opportunity for all group members to contribute, in some way, from the outset of the session. Ideas for icebreakers include:

1 Throwing a soft ball (preferably one that makes a funny noise when caught) around the circle, asking group members to say their name as they catch the ball. This activity is usually effective in raising a smile and acting as a reminder about names.

2 Asking group members in turn a closed question about themselves, for example: Where did you live as a child? What was your first job? Only use this icebreaker if you are confident that group members will be able to recall the answer easily. Ensure everyone has a turn in answering the question before prompting individuals to recall more detailed memories. This icebreaker is effective in giving everyone the opportunity to have a say at the outset of the group and may also reveal links between group members who have shared a common neighbourhood or occupation.

3 Pass a basket of small artefacts (triggers) representing the chosen theme for the session around the group, encouraging each member to take one item. In turn, ask each group member to say why they chose the item and if a memory is associated with it. Ensure there are sufficient objects for all the group members. If two members want the same item, encourage them to move together and share the object. This activity gives everyone a chance to share a memory at the beginning of the group.

4 Begin the session with well-remembered songs that individuals can sing along to together; encourage group members to link arms or hold hands while they sing. This icebreaker helps to promote a relaxed atmosphere and evoke memories through music.

Use of appropriate questions and responses.

- Try to avoid the use of the question: 'Do you remember…? or 'What do you remember about…?' Use more fail-proof alternatives: 'What does this remind you of?', or 'What do you think of when you look at this object?', 'It would be good to hear your memories about…' 'Do you remember?' questions can emphasize a lack of memory, and feelings of failure when individuals have to admit to difficulties in answering the question.

- Use open questions to encourage more detailed memories. For example 'What was your first or early days at school like?', 'How did you cope with a long walk to school in the winter?' Open questions encourage more detailed responses than closed questions, which usually provoke only one-word answers and do not allow for memories to be expanded, for example, 'Were you an only child?', or 'Did you have a happy or sad childhood?'

- Summarise an individual's contribution and ask if the comment reminded others of any memories. For example, 'Lorna has told us what it was like to get up early to do chores around the house before school. When did the rest of you do your chores?'

- Allowing sufficient time for individuals to respond to prompting questions and get in touch with memories is valuable. Older people express a lot of pleasure in being allowed the opportunity to get in touch with recollections that are not usually part of their familiar repertoire of memories.

MEDIATING AS GROUP LEADER

The promotion of a positive reminiscence experience for all group members may, at times, depend on the group leader's ability to mediate between individuals in the group. This may involve ensuring that no one individual monopolises group time with a long uninterrupted flow of memories, denying others the opportunity to share their recollections. Dominant group members often play the role of recall 'experts' (see Chapter 2), they have quick recall and often enjoy telling amusing stories from their past. Group leaders need to quieten dominant group members to avoid irritation growing within the group. Often, the group leader drawing in others is sufficient to remind the individual that they are part of a group process. However, if this is not successful it may be helpful to remind the individual of any group ground rules agreed about giving everyone a chance to share their memories. Continue by summarising the last memory the individual shared, turning towards others in the group to encourage their involvement.

Another difficult situation that involves mediation by the group leader is when one individual corrects another about the accuracy of their recall. It is vital that the group leader protects individuals from being devalued in this way. In this situation, it is important to emphasize that remembering is a very personal process and that the role of the group is to support each other and enjoy, not devalue, individuals' memories.

The use of racist or sexist language is another area that requires sensitive group mediation, particularly if it is aimed at a member of the group. It is essential that group leaders immediately make it clear that offensive comments are disrespectful and hurtful and cannot be tolerated.

MAKING ENDINGS SPECIAL

Endings are important events in the lifetime of reminiscence groups. Reminding group members each week how many sessions are left, and discussing ideas for making the last session special, helps group members prepare for the end of the group. The last session can be used, in part, to look back on what has been shared during the lifetime of the group; to plan for future groups; to prepare any display or publication about the memories shared in the group; or to share a group treat, for example, an outing to a local favourite place, a meal out, or preparing and eating together favourite traditional foods.

In looking back on what has been shared during the lifetime of the group, it is helpful to remind group members of the themes they particularly enjoyed, and any funny stories that were recounted. The last meeting is also an opportunity for group members to look at what they enjoyed or did not enjoy about the sessions.

SAVING MEMORIES

In the lifetime of a reminiscence group many interesting, entertaining and illuminating memories will be shared by a group of older people. It is valuable to decide as a group whether to save these memories for display or publication within the home, day setting or local community. Older people enjoy sharing their reminiscence experience with relatives, friends and carers. Additionally, seeing memories in print or on general display is a very positive and valuing message for older people.

Ideas for saving memories

- Photo board of group members looking at reminiscence objects or taking part in a reminiscence activity. A caption can be included, quoting group members' shared memories about the object or activity.
- Short booklet of group members' favourite recipes, poems or sayings.
- Newsletter about the reminiscence group, quoting group members' memories.
- Video of all or part of a group session.
- A temporary display of triggers used during the lifetime of the group, with quotes of group members' memories relating to each trigger.

THEME WEEKS

In addition to running group reminiscence sessions, many residential and day settings run reminiscence theme weeks: a theme is selected for one or two weeks, and over this period one or more communal areas are filled with triggers relating to the chosen theme. Residents, day-clients or patients are encouraged to visit the theme room and enjoy the artefacts, music and photographs. Staff, family and friends, community groups and local heritage museums, are often approached for the loan of items. These theme weeks allow a large number of older people to enjoy and be stimulated by the past. Additionally, theme weeks provide an opportunity to regularly change part of the everyday environment of older people, creating interest and a talking point.

SETTING UP REMINISCENCE ROOMS

Reminiscence rooms are a similar idea to theme weeks: a permanent space is dedicated to recreating one or more periods from the past (usually an era between the 1920s and 1940s). Decoration, furnishings, general artefacts, photographs and music, in the reminiscence room, match those of the era as closely as possible. These reminiscence rooms are ideal for use as venues for formal structured group or one-to-one reminiscence sessions, and informally, by individuals or groups of older people with the desire to relax in an atmosphere steeped in the past.

Eleanor Wilson, the manager of a psychiatric day hospital in Scotland, had been involved in a project to create a reminiscence room: a purpose-built room had been decorated and furnished in the style of the 1920s–1940s. The reminiscence room has a kitchen area, which includes artefacts donated by Scottish Television. All the staff on the unit were involved in planning the room and collecting appropriate furnishings. Eleanor Wilson (2000) writes with evident pleasure about the success of the room:

> Our reminiscence room has become one of our most valuable and best-used resources… Patients who have previously been quiet and withdrawn have been seen to become talkative and animated as they recount tales from their childhood.

Reminiscence room projects will hopefully become a more extensive resource in the future, providing large 'living' areas dedicated to acknowledging and celebrating the past. Older people in these atmospheric settings are stimulated to recall memories by being transported back to another era.

Summary Points

Running and Maintaining Reminiscence Groups

- The appropriate choice of themes and triggers brings a memories group to life. Themes that include a 'doing' element are particularly evocative in stirring memories.
- Triggers need to appeal to a variety of senses and be relevant to all cultures represented in groups.
- Use of icebreakers, open questions, summarising memories and mediation between group members promotes group communication.
- It is valuable to plan how to make a group's last session special.
- Saving and sharing memories values older people's histories.

5 Reminiscence Work and the Challenge of Dementia

As my grip on the present slips, more and more comfort is found within my memories of the past. DIANA FRIEL MCGOWIN, *Living in the Labyrinth*

This chapter looks at how the values, ideas and ways of working within a reminiscence-based approach respond to the challenge of dementia. Consideration is given to where the approaches described in the previous chapters need to be adapted or developed, to offer people with dementia a positive and enriching reminiscence experience.

At the cornerstone of the reminiscence approach to working with people with dementia is communication. 'Tuning in' and empathetically 'being with' the person with dementia builds communication links that help to maintain the uniqueness of individuals. Increasingly, good practice with people with dementia highlights the importance of focusing on characteristics, interests, skills, likes and dislikes that make up the uniqueness of individuals. A diagnosis of dementia with all its associated negative connotations, is viewed as secondary to the intrinsic value of an individual.

Kitwood and Bredin (1992) strongly support care practices for people with dementia that emphasize working with the uniqueness of individuals, believing that carers should be encouraged to be 'person-centred': looking at the whole person, rather than focusing narrowly on either individuals' difficult behaviour or decreasing abilities. The individuality of people with dementia is looked for, highlighted and maintained in care regimes that follow a person-centred approach.

Reminiscence work, with its ability to illuminate the past, provides opportunities for carers to respond creatively to individuals' histories and to acknowledge and value communication, in the present, about life themes from the past. Goldsmith *et al* (1997) highlight the value of communication with people with dementia:

> We believe that communication can be the key to unlocking past memories and discovering that 'there's life beyond the illness'.

DEVELOPING COMMUNICATION PATHS

Communication paths opened up with people with dementia, through the process of reminiscence work, are valuable in offering:

- An opportunity for the expression of long-held-on-to pain
- Reassurance, support and clarity about present situations
- Feelings of enjoyment and self-worth in revisiting positive past times

Much that is communicated by people with dementia in the present has links with people, roles, places and experiences from the past. Knowledge of, and insight into an individual's past can provide an understanding of repetitive requests, concerns and questions voiced in the present. Ways of responding may be indicated that are able to make a comfortable, secure link between the past and present for the person with dementia; as illustrated in the case of Ethel.

> Ethel, a widow in her eighties, living in a nursing home, regularly expressed concern that she had not seen George, her husband, for days. Ethel's carer had gained a lot of information about George from Ethel and her daughters. When Ethel became distressed about George, her carer would use information from the past to calm Ethel's present feelings: she would talk about George's job and the couple's life together.
>
> By taking this approach, Ethel was given the opportunity to get back in touch with her past by recalling comforting memories about her husband. George was always spoken of in the past tense, avoiding any collusion that he was still alive, but Ethel was not reminded about his death unless she referred directly to the event. After a time, Ethel would usually become calmer and the carer would suggest she came with her to help carry out one of the small domestic tasks that Ethel enjoyed.

Ethel's carer responded to her distress in the present by communicating via familiar and meaningful past memories. By renewing this positive link with the past, Ethel was helped to find a greater calmness in the present. A contrasting approach, often taken by carers when faced with a similar situation, is one that fails to engage the past in easing feelings in the present; individuals are often responded to pragmatically and given factual information about the death of a spouse. This response often results in the individual with dementia painfully reliving the grief of the loved one's death, as if it was the first time they had been told of the event.

Generally, it adds to an individual's distress, if when asking to see a deceased parent or spouse, they are constantly reminded of the loved one's death. The alternative approach of constructing effective communication paths with individuals based on positive memory links with the past enlists the power of personal history to ease distress in the present.

PLEASURE-IN-THE-MOMENT

People with dementia retain the ability to experience pleasure-in-the-moment; if carers have knowledge about what a person with dementia still enjoys doing, observing or being helped to accomplish, they are in a position to help individuals experience pleasure-in-the-moment. Additionally, the activity, interest or object that provided the pleasure-in-the-moment offers rich material for building communication paths between carer and the individual. Often pleasure-in-the-moment is derived from short, and possibly repetitive, activities that may be quickly forgotten by the individual. However, if a person with dementia gains enjoyment from an activity, the resulting enhanced mood may linger long after involvement in the activity has been forgotten.

Reminiscence work, with its ability to unlock information about the previous interests and preferences of an individual, provides ideas for creating pleasure-in-the-moment. Former interests may still be able to offer pleasure, albeit in a scaled-down form to fit in with the changed circumstance of individuals. For example, it may not be possible for an individual to continue to grow vegetables in an allotment, but pleasure may be gained in helping a carer to plant and look after a crop of garden tomatoes. In this, and similar ways, a person with dementia can be enabled to gain pleasure from a favourite pastime, resulting in an increased sense of purpose in the present. Reminders and encouragement will be needed to maintain interests, offering carers an opportunity to keep open a supportive communication path with the older person in the present.

Promoting pleasure-in-the-moment in the care of people with dementia helps to maintain individuality, increases generalised feelings of purpose and value, and builds links in the present between individuals and their carers.

THINKING POINT

Is there an older person you care for who has had to give up a favourite activity or interest due to recent or long-term difficulties? With support is there a way, even in a more limited form, that the particular interest could be resumed?

Reminiscence work with people with dementia helps carers foster care practices that are person- rather than illness- or problem-centred. By opening up many effective communication paths, reminiscence variously offers stimulation, comfort, purpose and familiarity to individuals. Working through this chapter will identify many more ideas for the creative use of reminiscence-based activities with people with dementia.

UNDERSTANDING DEMENTIA

A person-centred approach to the care of people with dementia emphasizes the person's personality, life history, remaining abilities, interests and responses to their present situation. However, adopting a person-centred approach to the care of older people with dementia does not remove the need to develop knowledge and awareness of dementia itself.

Initially, it is helpful to have a broad picture of the different conditions that result in a diagnosis of dementia; their prevalence and the existence of conditions that mimic dementia but may be only temporary illnesses. Dementia is a general term used to cover a group of diseases that have comparable impact on the brain and resultant effects on all functions of the mind. Dementia results in a progressive deterioration in reasoning, recall and self-help abilities; an individual's personality and behaviour may also succumb to the damaging effects of dementia. The rate and exact nature of deterioration in the functions mentioned will vary between individuals.

DISEASES CAUSING DEMENTIA

The largest proportion of people (approximately 50 per cent) diagnosed with dementia have *Alzheimer's disease*. This disease results in the greatest overall deterioration in an individual's functioning. It is not restricted to older people, individuals as young as 45 years old suffer from the disease. Some older people may have the disease for up to 10 years before it results in their death; other individuals die of another cause prior to the disease running its full course.

Vascular dementia accounts for the second largest number of people experiencing dementia. Some people have both Alzheimer's disease and vascular dementia. The latter is also known as *multi-infarct dementia* (MID) and *arteriosclerotic dementia*. Vascular dementia is triggered by strokes in the brain, and is marked by uneven deterioration in functioning, depending on the variable rate at which the brain experiences damage. A smaller number of people have dementia as a result of diseases such as *Lewy Body disease*, *Korsakoff's syndrome* (a dementia caused by alcohol abuse, which is non-progressive if treated), *Pick's disease*, *Creutzfeldt-Jakob disease* and HIV.

In the year 2000, the death of an older person, a 74-year-old man, was the first to be found attributable to Variant Creutzfeldt-Jakob disease, the human form of BSE found in cattle. In view of this finding doctors and scientists are now beginning to question how many older people may have been given an incorrect diagnosis for the cause of their dementia. This development is likely to have implications for the future diagnosing of dementia.

It is important to be aware that some illnesses and events in individuals' lives may result in the sudden onset of symptoms similar to those of dementia. These include infections, medication, reactions to bereavement, shock, depression, head injury, severe dehydration and hypothermia. Depression, in particular, may result in symptoms akin to those of dementia.

DEMENTIA – THE FACTS

(*Information Source*: Quiz Quest Game, Dementia Services Development Centre, University of Stirling.)

There are many misconceptions surrounding dementia. Decide which of the following statements are true or false:

- ***Statement 1***
  More people diagnosed as having dementia live in care establishments than at home or in the homes of members of their family.
  True or False?

- ***Statement 2***
  Approximately three out of five older people in their eighties are likely to have dementia.
  True or False?

- ***Statement 3***
  People with dementia take up to five times as long to respond to questions compared to people of the same age without dementia.
  True or False?

- ***Statement 4***
  Calling a person with dementia by their name each time you speak to them helps to maintain a sense of self.
  True or False?

How did it go? Check your choices below:

- ***Statement 1***
  This statement is false. Of the approximately 550,000 people in Britain with a diagnosis of dementia, around 80 per cent still live in their own home or with relatives.

- ***Statement 2***
  This statement is false. Approximately one, not three, in five of older people in their eighties have been diagnosed as having dementia.

- ***Statement 3***
  This statement is true, emphasising the need to think carefully about how we communicate effectively with older people with dementia.

- ***Statement 4***
  This statement is true. An individual's name is a significant part of their identity; the correct and regular use of an older person's name is an essential part of maintaining and promoting a sense of self.

A JOURNEY THROUGH DEMENTIA

The symptoms shown at different stages in the progress of dementia will vary between individuals. However, there are some areas of change in behaviour and thought patterns that are more likely to be experienced at onset of the disease, and others that are usually associated with the progressive stages.

It may be helpful to highlight one older person's journey through dementia, to illustrate the changes in behaviour, abilities and memory experienced during the different stages of dementia.

Bob, a widower in his late seventies, had lived with his wife Mary for 40 years before her death two years previously. Bob and Mary had two daughters who both lived locally. Mary's death, at home, had been sudden and a great shock to Bob. In the months prior to his wife's death, Bob had complained of increasing forgetfulness. He would often find himself at the local shops, totally at a loss as to what he had been intending to buy. Every decision or bill that needed paying became a major event for Bob, and he generally needed a great deal of reassurance to manage. Additionally, he was generally more anxious and restless than normal. Mary took over more and more of the tasks Bob would have easily accomplished previously. Bob regularly complained of 'not feeling himself', and was frustrated by what was happening to him.

In the months following their mother's death, Bob's daughters took turns in having their father to stay. With the trauma of their mother's death, both daughters forgot about their father's increasing agitation and forgetfulness prior to Mary's death. However, both were acutely aware of Bob's pain following his wife's death. He was at a loss without Mary, often physically looking for her in the house and street. Bob rarely mentioned Mary's death; usually spoke of his wife in the present tense, and would appear to be waiting for her to come back.

Initially, Bob's daughters viewed this searching behaviour as a normal part of bereavement, but when it continued for months both became concerned. Additionally, Bob would increasingly ask the same question repetitively. He began to lose all sense of time, not knowing what day of the week it was, even when reminded regularly. Bob would often seem to be living in the time of his early married life, in terms of both his conversations and behaviour. He would often want to get up very early to dress for work and ask where Mary was, particularly at mealtimes.

Concern led to Bob's doctor being consulted. He felt strongly that in view of the long-term and increasing nature of Bob's disorientation, together with the ongoing lengthy period of 'searching' for Mary, over six months after her death, he could be suffering from a disease resulting in symptoms of dementia. The doctor advised Bob's family that he would make a referral to a psychiatrist for a full specialist assessment.

Bob's detailed assessment by the specialist resulted in a diagnosis of Alzheimer's disease, possibly with a hastened progression as a result of the shock of the sudden death of his wife. Bob continued to live with his daughters over the following six months. An arrangement that became increasingly difficult due to Bob's growing disorientation. He started getting up several times at night, wanting to go out to work and repetitively asking where Mary was. Eventually both daughters could no longer cope with Bob's needs and their own families' demands, and he was admitted to a local residential home, nearly 18 months after Mary's death.

At the point of moving to residential care, Bob was showing clear signs of middle stage dementia, with disorientation to time and place, distressed searching behaviour for his dead wife, and regular persistent repetition of questions the answers to which he often forgot in seconds.

Bob's response to residential care; the progress of his dementia, and his involvement in group reminiscence work follows later in this chapter.

UNDERSTANDING AND RESPONDING TO COMMUNICATION

Reminiscence work with people with dementia, as it reveals personal histories, enhances carers' empathy. As a result, a more complete view of individuals develops, which in turn facilitates a personhood approach to caring.

Positive reminiscence work relies on effective communication skills as outlined in Chapter 2 – 'Promoting Reminiscence'. However, when working with people with dementia, enhanced skills and sensitivity must be 'bolted on' to these basic communication skills. Kitwood and Bredin (1992) strongly support the view that there is a need to develop special skills to communicate with people with dementia, and emphasize the importance of not relying on the literal meaning of words. It is essential to seek the underlying need or concern that prompt an individual's communication, in order to 'get a sense of the feeling that is coming across in the words'. Awareness of the factors that influence how people with dementia send and receive verbal and non-verbal messages plays an important role in increasing sensitivity to their special communication needs within the reminiscence process.

SUMMARY OF FACTORS THAT INFLUENCE HOW PEOPLE WITH DEMENTIA COMMUNICATE

- As disorientation grows, life in general becomes increasingly perplexing for people with dementia, creating an ongoing need for reassurance and increased security.

- Repetitive requests to see parents, or return to once familiar places, can be indicators of feelings of insecurity.
- Words do not always make literal sense when spoken or received by people with dementia, but tone of voice, gestures and facial expressions all retain the ability to communicate messages.
- People with dementia take up to five times longer to absorb and respond to information than people of the same age who are not experiencing dementia.
- Individuals for whom English is a second language will often revert to their mother tongue as their dementia advances.

WAYS OF ENHANCING COMMUNICATION WITH PEOPLE WITH DEMENTIA

- Ask short questions one at a time, rephrasing if an individual does not respond after some time.
- Show with gestures as well as words what you would like an individual to do.
- Show an individual the available choices, when asking to state a preference about clothing or meals.
- 'Tune in' to individuals' behaviour, feelings and facial expressions to increase understanding and empathy.
- Use reminiscence material about life history to make links with individuals' past, to lessen distress in the present.
- Use knowledge about past interests and likes to provide opportunities for creating pleasure-in-the-moment for individuals.
- Try to ask questions that do not emphasize a lack of memory. Instead of 'Do you remember?' try 'Does this remind you of anything?', or 'What does this make you think of?'
- Touch communicates caring. Try a hug, hand-holding or hand massage with oils.
- Listen with focused attention, and an open facial expression that communicates empathy and interest.
- Smiling and laughing with individuals helps to create an atmosphere of warmth and trust.
- Be aware of personal frustrations and fears in communicating with people with dementia. Develop personal strategies to cope with the demands of this kind of caring.

THINKING POINT

Is there an individual you care for with dementia whom you have recently found difficult to understand? Have the ideas on the enhancing communication list given you any new thoughts about how to work with this older person?

GROUPWORK

This section looks at how the basic points about running reminiscence groups (see Chapter 4) can be developed to promote a positive reminiscence experience for people with dementia. The main focus areas are size, timing, themes and triggers, and challenging communications.

Size

Small groups with only two to four members are appropriate for people with dementia. Two leaders are essential in order that all the members have sufficient attention to promote their involvement in, and enjoyment of, the reminiscence process.

Small groupwork affords people with dementia the opportunity to enjoy the general social atmosphere of being with peers. Joining in or watching reminiscence-based activities, such as listening to music, or helping to prepare and eat traditional dishes, provides pleasure and a stimulus to memory. A practical reminiscence-based activity, such as traditional food preparation, offers a shared, hands-on experience that provides sensory stimulation through touch, smell and taste.

One-to-one reminiscence work may at times seem more appropriate for individuals with dementia, particularly if they are restless in a group setting. However, restlessness in people with dementia can indicate a need to be involved in more meaningful activities. Interaction with peers in a reminiscence group, even where there is diminished ability to clearly follow conversations clearly, may provide a welcome change for an otherwise socially isolated individual.

Group reminiscence work can be enhanced for individuals by the increase of background history gained through one-to-one work. Background history enables a more personally relevant approach to the selection of themes and triggers in groupwork. Personal relevance of reminiscence cues is vital in working with people with dementia, to facilitate their recall of memories.

Timing

Sessions need to be short, approximately 20 minutes and frequent if possible, at least twice a week. Choose a time of day when the group members are most at ease and least disorientated. The same venue and time of day for each session creates a familiar routine. Including a break for refreshments, even when running short sessions, helps to create a relaxed group atmosphere.

Themes and triggers

Within the reminiscence process when working with people with dementia, it is essential to focus on identifying themes that have significant individual meaning for group members. Reminiscence 'research' with individuals, family members and friends, during the preparatory stages of the group, provides background information that aids the selection of personally relevant reminiscence cues.

Personal information gathered about group members may highlight one or more themes that hold common interest for the group. For example, all the group members may have worked in shops at some point in their lives; a general theme for a session could be 'work', with individual triggers being obtained that would act as a reminiscence cue for each group member. These triggers could include photographs of the kind of shop each member worked in; objects similar to those sold in the different shops; old style scales and weights used at the time, or pre-decimal money.

The value and enjoyment that can be gained by individuals when time and effort is taken to discover personally relevant themes and triggers is illustrated in Nora's reminiscence experience.

> Nora had worked in a grocer's shop as a young girl, and one of the memories she had often talked about in the past with her family was being faced with a huge block of butter and being asked to cut it into one pound shapes. In a reminiscence session where the theme was 'work', Nora had eagerly picked up a pair of old wooden butter pats and smilingly began to mime their use in shaping butter. Nora, as in previous sessions, did not take part verbally in the group, but her non-verbal response to a personally significant trigger clearly showed enjoyment and engagement in the reminiscence process.

When working with people with dementia, it is important to recognise the value of all responses to the process of reminiscing, whatever form they take and however momentary.

Music

Music is an invaluable trigger for recall and enjoyment when working with people with dementia in small group reminiscence sessions. One of the skills retained for the longest in people with dementia is the ability to remember and sing-along to familiar songs of the past. Even when everyday speech has been affected by strokes and/or dementia, individuals are often able to take part in sing-alongs. Using reminiscence 'research' to discover each individual's favourite singers, or kinds of music, will add to the power of chosen music to evoke memories. Additionally, the togetherness of general group responses to music such as singing, clapping, holding hands and swaying, all promote a positive atmosphere in which to share memories.

Playing or listening to music contributed greatly to the past lives of many older people, and can offer an invaluable trigger in recall when working with people with dementia.

THINKING POINT

Can you think of anyone you have cared for with dementia for whom one song or piece of music is particularly evocative? Do you know, or could you find out, why this particular music has meaning for them?

Aromas

Triggers that appeal to the sense of smell can be particularly evocative to people with dementia. A once-familiar smell can transport individuals back to a well-remembered time or event. The smell of a rose; fish and chips in newspaper; moth balls; home-made baking; applying and smelling a little 'Lily of the Valley' or '4711' perfume from an original scent bottle, and many other smells can help evoke memories. The more pertinent the aroma is to the individual the greater the impact it will have as a reminiscence cue.

The role played by smell in recall is fully appreciated in China: important family events are marked by talking about them in a group, while passing around a pot of strong-smelling herbs. The belief is that years later the smell of the herbs will powerfully evoke the event.

The use of aromatherapy with people with dementia is a growing area and one that focuses on the senses of touch and smell. It involves the use of massage with essential oils to communicate valuing, comfort and attention. The smell of the oils has the power to enhance and change moods making this a skilled way of working with people, which requires specialised training. However, hand massage with basic oils requires no formal training and is an excellent way of offering individuals relaxing and valuing attention.

Bob and the themes of his life

Reminiscence 'research' carried out with Bob and his family on his admission to residential care proved invaluable in identifying themes and triggers that were to enliven his experience of group reminiscence.

Bob often spoke and acted as if he had returned to the time when he was a young working man still living with his parents. The theme of work therefore seemed an ideal one on which to base initial reminiscence 'research'. Bob could recall many memories about his own early working life in a bank. However, the memories that gave him the most pleasure were those about his father's job as a signalman on the local railway. This reminded Bob's daughters of their father's love of model railways, and how at one time he had had a railway layout in the loft. Bob smiled as they talked of his love of everything to do with railways.

The information gained from this reminiscence 'research' with Bob and his family, stimulated many ideas about appropriate and personally relevant multi-sensory triggers connected with the themes of work and railways:

- Sound recordings of train whistles and trains leaving stations
- Photographs of stations, signal boxes, old steam trains
- Old train timetables
- Loan of a model railway from a local museum, family, friends, staff, or an enthusiast in the community

Coping with troubled communication.

The impact of dementia on memories, and the potential they hold to provoke troubled communication in the present will vary, but often includes the following:

- Progressive erosion of memory store, initially affecting short-term memory, and subsequently recall of the more distant past.

- Painful, unresolved feelings from the past increasingly being recalled.

- A highlighting of the times in individuals' lives when they felt purposeful and needed.

- Reduced ability to understand reasons that can force a change in personal living situations.

- Disorientation caused, in part, by the splintering of short-term memory, creating insecurity and a lack of familiarity in the present, resulting in individuals longing to return to the time when they had the security of the love of parents or other childhood carers.

As a result of the effects of dementia on memory and perception of the present, communications often arise in reminiscence sessions that are difficult or painful to handle, both for the individual with dementia and the reminiscence worker.

Pain and the past

Recall of the past can evoke positive and negative feelings: painful memories can arise at any point in the process of remembering. Individual memories often link to form a chain of recall about a specific time, event or relationship in an individual's life, creating the potential for a mixture of happy and sad recall during reminiscence sessions. Bob's experience in reminiscence sessions at his residential home clearly illustrates this potential for happy and sad recall.

> From Bob's pleasurable response in recalling memories around the theme of railways, it was clear how much enjoyment and relaxation this particular reminiscence communication path opened up for Bob. Unfortunately, Bob's pleasure in this link with the past was often short-lived; even when apparently immersed in happy memories he would suddenly start asking about his wife and when she would return. Bob would look very sad and lost in these moments.
>
> To support Bob during these distressing times of sad recall, Bob's carer began building a reminiscence communication path focusing on Bob's life with his wife. Subsequently, when Bob asked for his wife, his carer responded in a way that allowed Bob to express the sadness he felt at that moment, offering comfort by touching or holding his hand. Additionally, Bob's carer had learned a great deal about Mary from his daughters, and knew the memories he particularly liked to be prompted to recall about their life together.
>
> Bob's carer always referred to his wife in the past tense, to avoid any collusion with Bob's belief that he would see Mary again. Bob usually appeared easier after expressing his sadness and having the opportunity to talk about Mary, thus renewing a link with a positive time in his past.

Pain in remembering may be experienced and expressed, during or outside reminiscence sessions, while recalling prompted or unprompted memories about a time in the past. Individuals may express their pain in the form of repetitive demands to once again see parents, a dead partner or child. In an attempt to overcome this distress, a wish or need may be stated, often at the same time each day, to go to work or back home to look after parents or children. Through these painful communications, arising from recall of the past, people with dementia may be sending out messages to carers to show that they were once needed and purposeful people, living in close, loving relationships. They may be reminding themselves and their carers that they still need to have a role in life, and a sense of purpose with opportunities to care and be cared for.

At times, in group sessions, being faced with individuals' pain about past and present situations may feel overwhelming to carers. However, although every individual is different and the causes of distress variable, there are some strategies that generally help:

- 'Being with' the person, as they express verbally or non-verbally their distress without rushing in with assurances and distractions; touching or holding an individual's hand if that is a known comfort to them.

- Acknowledging and valuing the person, time of life or activity that the individual is missing. Helping with information gained in reminiscence 'research', to renew a comforting, positive memory link with the past.

Encouraging the individual to linger with, and expand the memory, if this eases the distress.

- What is it that offers this individual pleasure-in-the-moment? Is there an activity they would enjoy taking part in, which would offer pleasure and a sense of purposefulness? Depending on individual preferences, ideas for providing pleasure-in-the-moment include an accompanied walk around the home or garden; hand massage with oils; stroking a loved pet, or helping with a favourite domestic task.

As dementia progresses, it is more difficult for individuals to realistically evaluate their lives or avoid dwelling on painful recall. Additionally, people with dementia may have little or no understanding about why certain life changes have happened, for example, there are often generalised feelings of loss and hopelessness expressed when remembering a former home.

During group reminiscence sessions, individuals may share concern about events that happened in childhood or young adulthood. Recall associated with these life stages may be frequent and intense. Memories of distressing events that have lain dormant for many years may suddenly come to the surface forcing the individual to confront painful feelings. If, when faced with this situation, the reminiscence worker can remain calm, confident and attentive, individuals will feel accepted and able to express their distress. Repetition of painful feelings associated with a past event may be an invaluable way for individuals to complete 'grief work', unfinished or denied in the past. Each repetition, particularly if received with empathetic responses, may ultimately provide an opportunity for individuals to let go of long-term emotional pain.

THINKING POINT

Are you caring for someone with dementia who is facing the pain of past losses, or other distressing events that happened in their younger days? What form does this distress take? How are you managing to help the individual? Which of the strategies described may help to lessen the person's distress?

If reminiscence workers are able to 'be with' people with dementia in their pain, not leaving them to struggle alone with overwhelming feelings from long ago, opportunities exist to ease distress. Equally, if we are able to provide some clarity and reassurance to counter individuals' disorientation about why they are in their present living situation, feelings of loss often experienced by people with dementia may be eased.

Reminiscence work has value in the lives of people with dementia, not only for the role it can play in accompanying individuals through their painful memories, but also in the opportunity it provides to transport them back to a time when they felt purposeful and needed. Robert Davis (1993) succinctly sums up the value that this latter attribute of reminiscence work holds for him:

> Blessed is the person who can take an Alzheimer's patient back to that happier time when they were worthwhile and allow them to see the situation in which they were of some use.

Coping with troubled communications in reminiscence groups is one of the key skills needed by group leaders and involves, in part, an acceptance of the mixed emotional nature of recall for many people with dementia.

PROMOTING A PROGRAMME OF REMINISCENCE-BASED ACTIVITIES

The provision of a programme of daily reminiscence-based activities promotes groupwork with people with dementia by offering a purposeful and enjoyable routine for individuals and their carers. Individuals experiencing different stages of dementia may be included in a reminiscence-based programme: some will enjoy taking part in activities, while others will experience pleasure and stimulation from being with peers in a warm atmosphere.

The potential value of reminiscence-based programmes of daily activities for people with dementia is supported by the findings of a study undertaken by Rovner *et al* (1990). The study followed up two groups of individuals, at comparable stages in their dementia, living in nursing-home settings with similar staffing levels. One group lived in a dementia unit that offered a programme of activities for up to 40 hours a week, while the second lived in a unit with activities for only three to five hours a week. The follow-up after a year showed that only two people in the first group, with an extensive activity programme, showed signs of further deterioration, compared with nine in the unit with a far more limited programme.

A general daily programme of reminiscence-based activities can be developed to suit individuals, their carers and the needs of the unit. For people in the more progressive stages of dementia, being in a group setting can feel secure, if there are sufficient numbers of carers to allow time for regular one-to-one attention. Feelings of isolation and loneliness may be lessened, even for individuals who are finding it increasingly difficult to follow general conversation. If an atmosphere of warmth and acceptance exists within the group, individuals will sense a feeling of being valued. Where the majority of people in a unit are in the later stages of dementia, reminiscence-based activities can be developed that have an emphasis on quiet, sensory involvement for individuals and carers. For example, the use of hand massage with oil, accompanied walks in the garden to smell or pick flowers, or listening together to music.

A reminiscence-based daily programme of activities proved beneficial to Bob as his dementia advanced:

Immediately following his admission to care, Bob had been helped, through the building of reminiscence communication paths, to renew interests from the past and gain comfort over the loss of his wife. However, Bob's dementia advanced steadily to the point where he could not recognise his daughters, causing them great distress. His recall of the past now centred almost totally on his life as a boy, and he would regularly ask for his father. Mary, his wife, would be pointed to in photographs and referred to as his mother. He needed help to eat and drink and go to the toilet. Bob would attempt to dress himself, but put clothes on in the wrong order and often back to front. He now gained the greatest comfort from being physically close to his carers, often following them about until they could sit with him. Bob continued to sense that his daughters cared for him, but could no longer acknowledge their relationship to him. Bob enjoyed his daughters' visits, during which he would sit holding their hands and smiling.

Bob was moved to a unit in the home for individuals in the progressive stage of dementia. The unit ran a daily programme of reminiscence-based activities that it was felt Bob would enjoy. He was very happy to be with others and settled when a carer was able to sit with him. Bob enjoyed the comfort of a hand massage and listening to familiar songs activities that were both part of the daily programme in the unit.

The following is an example of a programme of reminiscence-based activities that could be used to work with people with dementia on a daily basis.

Getting together

Initially, encourage individuals to sit together in a circle. Prompt individuals to throw a soft ball to each other, and as each person catches it, encourage them to say their name. An alternative getting-together activity involves going around the group, saying hello to everyone by name and reminding each individual about one object or interest that you are aware gives them pleasure:

> 'Hello Constance, I like the way you enjoy walking around the garden with me, smelling all the flowers.'
>
> 'Hello, Bill, I enjoy listening with you to songs by your favourite singer, Frank Sinatra.'

Flowers

An enjoyable group activity is looking at, smelling and arranging garden or wild flowers in an old-style vase or other container. This often provokes discussion about favourite flowers or gardening generally.

Music

Play one of a selection of appropriate sing-along tapes of old music, encouraging people to join in by singing, clapping or foot tapping. People usually enjoy about 10 minutes or more of this activity. Short extracts from well-known songs are the most successful. Compiling a tape with individuals' favourite songs is also particularly effective in promoting the greatest group involvement. Encourage the group to hold hands for the last song, to promote a feeling of togetherness.

Completing old sayings

Repeat the beginning of well-known sayings, asking the group to finish them for you. Many people with dementia continue to recall easily sayings they were familiar with in their childhood. They also enjoy hearing again sayings that appear to contradict each other. It will quickly become obvious which selection of sayings has the most meaning to individuals and is the easiest to complete.

Refreshments

Making and sharing a cup of tea together, at any point during the day, can be turned into a reminiscence-based activity by adopting the traditional way of making a pot of tea using a crock teapot, tea leaves, tea strainer and china teacups. Group discussion can be prompted by asking for advice about 'warming the pot'; how much loose-leaf tea to use; how long to leave the tea to brew, and whether a cup of tea made with loose-leaf tea tastes better than one made from tea bags. Carers sitting down with a group to enjoy a traditionally made cup of tea, or any other refreshments, promote a relaxed and sharing atmosphere. For a change, include a favourite traditional cake or other food that group members recall enjoying.

Hand massage

Giving individuals a hand massage with oils promotes a quiet relaxed atmosphere. The one-to-one attention offers reassurance and valuing, together with an opportunity for carers to pick up on how an individual is feeling about their present situation in the group. If a group member indicates that they do not want a hand massage, stay with the individual for a time, so that they do not miss out on the one-to-one attention.

Time for memories

Including a time when triggers associated with specific themes are used to evoke memories can be an integral part of a reminiscence-based programme. As emphasized previously, using themes and triggers specific to individuals' backgrounds offers the greatest impact on memory for people with dementia.

However, when working with a large group of up to six or eight members, it may be necessary to use triggers relating to a broad reminiscence theme to prompt memories, or for individuals to enjoy looking at or holding. This more general, less personalised approach to themes and triggers may suit some individuals who do not want to take part in the more intense, individualised atmosphere of recall. Try to use triggers that appeal to a number of senses, for variety and to offer sensory stimulus.

Memories in action

This activity provides the opportunity to encourage individuals to take part in a hands-on group task associated with interests or tasks from the past. Group hands-on activities could include cleaning brasses, darning socks, using a treadle sewing machine, or planting bulbs or seeds in pots. Individuals can be encouraged to actively take part in the hands-on activity or be involved by watching others. The physical doing of a task associated with the past can be a highly successful way of promoting recall and reminding individuals of skills they retain. Avoid stereotyped gender-based assumptions about which sex is likely to be interested in a particular hands-on activity.

Preparing a traditional dish or cake using old recipes and equipment can be a valuable hands-on activity; practical involvement in taking turns to stir, roll or mix ingredients, offering advice or simply watching others, provides a purposeful process, which helps to stimulate memories. In addition, sensory stimulus is provided by the look, smell and taste of the dish or cake.

Sharing a meal

Generally sitting together as a group, with carers, for a meal or part of a meal, promotes a sharing warm atmosphere. Encouraging individuals to help in laying the table prior to a meal and clearing and washing up afterwards, allows them to maintain feelings of purposefulness and retain some of their past domestic interests. Individuals, including those with mobility difficulties, are often able to help in some way with support and time. It is also possible for individuals to help wash and dry up, fold tablecloths, and lay up tables while sitting.

Relaxing together

Quiet, relaxing periods need to be incorporated into the daily programme, particularly following busy hands-on activities. Additionally, sensitivity to individuals makes it possible to recognise when someone has tired of a particular activity and needs a break. Many people find gardens relaxing, either to sit and overlook, or to walk or sit in with others. Many individuals also enjoy being helped to pick flowers. Being in a room where individuals can watch visitors coming and going, or traffic passing, can offer interest and a talking point. For some people with dementia this may be disorientating, as unsettled feelings are promoted about why they are not going home, or why a special person has failed to visit.

The above provides a selection of ideas for a reminiscence-based programme of daily activities. There are many other possible activities that could be included, depending on individuals' and carers' interests and skills. Different seasons, festivals and other traditional celebrations also provide ideas for activities to include in a daily programme of activities.

Reminiscence-based programmes offer a purposeful and valuing way of structuring social care for people with dementia; and carers giving time and commitment to empathetically 'being with' individuals is as important as the choice of activities. Individuals are able to take part in reminiscence-based programmes in a way that suits their needs and interests: they may want, with assistance, to take part in all or some of the activities; to watch and/or offer advice about how things were done in the past, or just be in a relaxed atmosphere with others. Memories may be stirred and shared in some instances; at other times, simply being around triggers, touching or holding the objects, may offer pleasure.

Whatever the impact of dementia is on individuals, the uniqueness of their life histories remains a crucial part of who they are. When approaching individuals about taking part in reminiscence work, on a group or one-to-one basis, sensitivity is needed to the individual's verbal and non-verbal indications as to how they feel generally about remembering. Additionally, ongoing sensitivity is required to observe and respond to varying day-to-day and longer-term attitudes to remembering. As dementia progresses it may change both the inclination to take part in recall and the emphasis of remembering for individuals.

Summary Points

Reminiscence and the Challenge of Dementia

- Enhanced listening and responding skills are valuable in the process of understanding the unique communication of each individual with dementia.
- One of the keys to positive reminiscence work with people with dementia is the building of communication paths, which respond to individuals' verbal and non-verbal messages about past and present situations.
- Knowledge and insight gained through reminiscence work helps to establish a person-centred approach to caring that emphasizes the uniqueness of individuals.
- By utilising information gained through reminiscence 'research', pleasure-in-the-moment can be promoted for individuals, providing enjoyment, interest and enhanced feelings of purpose and value.
- Themes and associated triggers that hold a sensory and personalised appeal to people with dementia are the most effective in prompting the recall of memories.
- Both regular small-group reminiscence sessions and daily group reminiscence-based activity programmes offer people with dementia and their carers a valuable social experience.

6 Reminiscence Work Across Cultures

Jamaica, he thought, was just Britain in the sun. ANDREA LEVY, *This is my England*

This chapter looks at how to effectively promote the inclusion of older people from minority cultures in sensitive one-to-one, and group reminiscence work.

The concept of culture in contemporary society has taken on a broad meaning that encompasses a number of characteristics common to the lives of a particular group of people: characteristics that include race, political and religious beliefs, family values and attitudes, and leisure habits. Sensitive reminiscence work with older people from minority cultures requires carers to acknowledge, value and celebrate diverse cultural backgrounds that embody life histories, religious beliefs and rituals, traditional celebrations and customs.

Carers working with older people from cultural backgrounds that differ from their own may be concerned that the lack of shared commonality of experience in terms of country of birth, language, family values, religious or traditional customs, creates a barrier to understanding. This concern may result in a lack of confidence about how to set about planning an appropriate reminiscence experience for people from minority cultures. There are valuable ways for carers to confront these concerns: acknowledgement and a willingness to overcome these reactions is the first step; finding out information about the cultural background of older people from individuals, books and documentaries; and developing an understanding of how British politics, past and present, including immigration and asylum laws, have affected the lives of older people from a range of cultures.

It is particularly important to appreciate the impact of emigration on people from minority cultures, on arrival in Britain, over the years and in the present as an older person. People from all minority cultures moving to a new homeland will have been exposed to both contrasting and similar experiences, feelings and reactions as the result of being a stranger a long way from home. Many people will have been shocked and hurt at being subjected to racism or religious intolerance. Reminiscence workers will need to be prepared to hear negative comments about how older people were and are treated in Britain as the direct result of belonging to a minority culture.

Devaluing incidents and attitudes will have been part of the experience of many people emigrating to Britain, whatever their circumstances, including those positively encouraged to leave their homeland in British colonies to come to the 'mother country', and refugees fleeing from war or persecution. Andrea Levy (2000) describes her parents' experience as immigrants in Britain in the late 1940s. In this post-war period, emigration to Britain from the West Indies and other countries was high. Andrea Levy highlights the overt racism faced by African-Caribbean people, and immigrants from many other countries, in finding work and accommodation. One example of overt racism she cites is a notice that graphically illustrates widely held attitudes of the day:

NO NIGGERS, NO DOGS, NO IRISH

Such instances were viewed by immigrants from minority cultures as shocking and disappointing: emigration to the 'mother country' had been portrayed as a chance for people from British colonies to make a new home in a country that would offer both a welcome and equality for all. Racism in many forms, overt and covert, formed the backdrop to the lives of people from minority cultures throughout their adjustment to the demands of work and family in a new homeland. Some incidents of racism would have been personal in nature; others degraded minority cultures generally; potentially, all were demeaning and hurtful, demanding a resilience to bear and overcome.

Today, older people from minority cultures within residential or day-care settings may experience a lack of awareness towards their cultural needs and practices. Care regimes, particularly when an older person is in a small minority within a home or day unit, may not fully reflect likes and customs surrounding particular foods or methods of cooking, celebration of culturally related festivals, or the observance of certain religious practices.

Reminiscence workers, in making a commitment to increase understanding and interest in minority cultures, create a climate for the growth of respectful, anti-discriminatory practice. Care patterns can be developed and enhanced that more closely reflect the needs of individuals from minority cultures. Additionally, being culturally aware heightens sensitivity to the need to challenge any discriminatory comments that arise in reminiscence groups. In instances where there is the use of inappropriate language it will be important to emphasize that the use of discriminatory stereotypes and language are not acceptable.

THINKING POINT

Think about one or more stereotypical comments you have heard about people from a minority culture. How do you react personally to the comment, or think an older person from the culture being stereotyped would react?

VALUE OF REMINISCENCE WORK

Working in a reminiscence way with people from minority cultures makes potentially enriching demands on carers, and offers great value to older people:

- Individuals are helped to establish, maintain or renew links with the culture of their original homeland, which is an enriching process for carers and individuals alike. Opportunities are created to enliven everyday life through, for example, the marking and celebration of traditional festivals.

- Many individuals take pride in their 'mother tongue', and reminiscence work that promotes the use of older people's first language, in both spoken and written form, helps to maintain this important element of cultural identity.
- Individuals may reclaim or increase pride and interest in their country of origin as a result of a respectful and sensitive approach shown towards their homeland.
- Opportunities are created for individuals to share their varying experiences in adopting a new land as their home, including any negative experiences arising from initial or ongoing racist attitudes shown by the majority culture. As a result, carers are able to share in a living history of how life was, and is, for older people who adopted Britain as a new homeland.
- Older people can be helped to acknowledge and applaud their success in having adapted to the demands of a new culture.
- Cultural history, traditions and rituals can be transmitted to younger generations through the written or sound recording of older people's memories. In this way young and old alike are enabled to feel a cultural continuity between the past, present and future.

CULTURAL BELIEFS AND ATTITUDES THAT INFLUENCE REACTIONS TO RECALL

An individual's cultural beliefs and attitudes may be a strong influence on their response to reminiscence work; different attitudes to being old, dying, death and grieving exist between cultures. Additionally, the willingness and interest older people have in sharing their past may vary between cultures. For example, the emphasis of reminiscence work in focusing on the past may be seen as a Western cultural approach, and may not appeal to a more present-orientated view adopted by some cultures. How life successes are measured and celebrated will also differ, with Eastern cultures generally taking a less individualised approach than Western cultures.

Reminiscence work that focuses on bereavement experiences may also evoke differing responses between cultures. Cultural customs to do with dying and death greatly affect how the experience of loss is coped with. For example, the traditional Western view of quiet, controlled grieving, contrasts strongly with the practice of some South-East Asian cultures, where more open expressions of distress are viewed as normal. Whatever cultural rituals and supports are available to individuals, it is important to remember that the tasks and feelings of grieving and grief are similar across cultures. It is the way that individuals show their loss and are helped to pass through and recover from bereavement which differ between cultures. Lendrum and Syme (1994) highlight the similarities in the feelings of loss across cultures:

> Different social networks and different cultural groups deal with grief in different ways. Whatever the rituals, however, the emotions of loss and disturbance are much the same.

Ensuring that personal wishes about cultural rituals prior to death, at the point of death and after death, are known and respected, help the dying to face death, and the bereaved in their grieving. Rituals that help individuals achieve a 'good death' vary according to religious or cultural beliefs. For example, followers of Islam may wish to face south-east, towards Mecca, as they are dying; practising Hindus may wish to lie on the floor prior to death; many religions believe in the importance of having prayers, scriptures or hymns recited to the dying by family members or religious leaders.

Many religions have strong beliefs about who should handle a body after death. Often only family members or members of the same religious faith are permitted to touch the body. Where family members are not available, or are unable to perform this task, workers need to adhere to the strict requirements of the particular culture or religion, to show respect for the body and the bereaved family.

Older people, depending on their religious and cultural beliefs, may have strong traditions related to mourning practices that have helped them come to terms with death in the past; adherence to these practices may continue to offer support in the face of loss in the present.

Within each religion and culture there are wide variations in the degree of belief and observance by individuals of traditional rituals related to dying, death and mourning. It is vital to talk to the individual and family members about their personal beliefs, views and wishes. Where family members are not available, community and/or religious leaders should be approached for advice.

Older people may or may not continue to experience fully the influences of their cultural origins. Additionally, where original cultural traditions and beliefs remain dominant in an older person's life, there will inevitably have been some assimilation of Western cultural influences. In many instances, older people may be coming to terms with their children and grandchildren adopting an increasingly Westernised approach to life. In terms of care of elders, focus by extended families on a Westernised approach to the care of older people may be at odds with how individuals had foreseen the role of their family. Reminiscence work in such situations may involve painful comparisons about how cultural beliefs about the traditional role played by older people in families have changed over time.

Promoting the personhood of individuals from minority cultures within the reminiscence process involves, in part, the acknowledgment that background culture has a varying emphasis and role in people's past and present lives.

REMEMBERING EMIGRATION

Emigrating to Britain and adapting to a new homeland will have been experienced uniquely by each individual, depending on factors such as their personality, previous life events, family support systems, health, housing and employment opportunities. However, through this diversity of experience of emigration run common threads of feelings, expectations and reactions, both within individual cultures and transculturally. The sharing, in group reminiscence, of both the commonalities and differences about such a major, life-changing event as emigration, has the potential to form links between older people from the same and different minority cultures.

The potential for transcultural empathy around the theme of emigration is illustrated in the reaction of minority cultural audiences to the Age Exchange Theatre production *Routes*, which was based on the experience of Asian elders who had emigrated to Britain. Their real-life stories were re-enacted through the play's portrayal of one young man's experiences on leaving India for the 'mother country' and subsequently growing old in Britain. The play highlighted the typical experiences and reactions encountered by immigrants in a new homeland, and the adaptations required to cope with unfamiliar environments. *Routes* played to audiences from many minority cultures in Britain and Europe: all empathised, often being moved to tears and laughter, over the commonality of experience and feelings shared with the British Asian elders.

THINKING POINT

Have you had the opportunity to discuss with an older person from a minority culture their hopes when they arrived in Britain as an immigrant? Did they share with you to what extent these hopes have been realised?

The commonalities and differences emanating from the experience of emigration provide potent material for reminiscence work, both in groups and on a one-to-one basis. Reminiscence workers need to be aware of how to respond to memories about emigration that may provoke painful and lasting feelings of regrets. As older people from minority cultures age, there may be a wish to be helped to re-evaluate the decision to emigrate: a decision that may have been unavoidable due to war, ethnic cleansing or economic plight, or a positive voluntary decision to move to a new homeland.

Some individuals may want to 'let go' of an original dream that carried them to Britain: many who emigrated did so believing they would one day return permanently to live in their original homeland. For other, older people, members of their extended family may have died before earlier promises could be honoured to pay for them to come to Britain. This may have resulted in lingering feelings of having let down family members, and possibly regrets about not being present when a loved one died. Feelings of survivor's guilt may be an issue for some older people who experienced war or natural disaster, but escaped while family and friends suffered or died.

It is important to retain a strong sense of people's individuality and uniqueness of experience even if there is a shared first language between reminiscence worker and individuals from minority cultures. Gibson (1998) considers this point, stressing that it is important not to assume that reminiscing with one minority cultural group will be easier than with another on the basis of being able to communicate in the same first language:

> Shared language obviously helps but many other subtle factors are also important.

For older people who emigrated to Britain from English-speaking countries such as Ireland or the Caribbean, there would have been as many issues and feelings around leaving their homeland and settling in Britain as for individuals who did not speak English as a first language.

PROMOTING INCLUSITIVITY

Reminiscence workers who are able to illustrate a heightened awareness of, and sensitivity to, the impact of the complex experience of emigration, and the role of cultural influences in the lives of individuals, develop increased empathy for people from minority cultures. In addition to illustrating increased awareness and sensitivity for older people from minority cultures, there are a number of practical factors to take into account when promoting their inclusion in positive one-to-one and group reminiscence work.

Language barriers

Overcoming possible exclusion of individuals from either one-to-one or group reminiscence experience due to difficulties in communication is vital. This may be a particular issue where individuals from different minority cultures are under-represented in a day- or residential setting.

Leaders of reminiscence groups should ideally be representative of the culture(s) of the group members present. Similarly, in one-to-one work there may be a greater willingness to take part in the reminiscence process if there is a shared minority cultural background between worker and older person. Conversely, factors other than cultural background may influence how well a worker is accepted by older people when undertaking reminiscence work. An individual may get on particularly well with a worker who does not originate from their minority culture, gaining enjoyment from the process of 'teaching' the individual about a different cultural experience.

Where leaders are not representative of the minority cultures of the group members, the use of interpreters may be vital to avoid language being a barrier to inclusion. Additionally, community nurses, social workers or volunteers from the local community, who share the same first language as group members, may be able to offer short-term involvement in reminiscence groups.

Offering the opportunity for people from minority cultures to share personal histories in their first language shows acknowledgement of and respect for the role played by language in cultural background, past and present. In addition, where individuals are experiencing dementia they may revert to communicating only in their first language, regardless of their previous level of spoken English. Invitations to, and posters about reminiscence events may need to be prepared in a number of languages, to reflect the first language of the individuals attending.

Where a group or individual decision is made to record memories for display, publication or private record only, it is important that there is an opportunity to choose whether memories are written in English, the first language of group members, or both. Retaining written memories in the first language of minority cultures communicates respect and valuing for the cultural background of individuals. Such recordings help to both transmit the content of memories and keep minority languages alive.

Many older people have a great desire to promote the learning of their first language by younger generations; enjoyment is often expressed in hearing the 'mother tongue' spoken by children and grandchildren. This desire of older people to transmit the value of their culture, in part through the speaking of their first language, is illustrated in *A Place to Stay* (Schweitzer, 1997). Here one older woman, who emigrated to England from India, sums up commonly expressed sentiments of concern about grandchildren not being taught the 'mother tongue' of previous generations as well as English:

> 'They are very young, they do not speak Punjabi. I always ask my children that they should teach them Punjabi, otherwise they will forget their culture, and when they go to India it will be hard for them, not to understand their mother tongue.'

By promoting the speaking of the first language of minority cultures during the reminiscence process, and recording memories in the 'mother tongue', cultural identity is strengthened and communicated to younger generations.

CO-WORKING

As discussed previously, co-working in the leadership of reminiscence groups is invaluable in offering older people an optimum reminiscence experience. The value of joint over sole leadership, together with the issues involved in co-working, were looked at in detail in Chapter 3. The comments in this earlier chapter, which relate to joint leadership in groupwork are also applicable when working with people from minority cultures.

However, group leaders working with minority cultures have several additional cultural-specific issues to consider, including:

- Is the group to be made up of a mix of older people from the white majority and minority culture(s) represented in the unit?
- If the group membership is to be culturally mixed are we, as prospective joint leaders, representative of both the majority and minority culture?
- As leaders from a minority and the white majority culture what issues do we need to think about in terms of our working relationship that leaders from a shared culture would not?

Factors that promote a sensitive reminiscence experience for a group membership of different cultural backgrounds include:

1. Co-leadership of the group with leaders representing the majority and minority cultural backgrounds of the group members.
2. The co-leader from the majority culture has background knowledge of the older people from the minority culture in the group.
3. The co-leader from the majority culture has an awareness of the potential effects of past and present personal and societal racism experienced by the older people from the minority culture in the group.
4. Group members from the different cultures being equally willing to show interest in each other's background and experiences.
5. Co-leaders apportioning roles and tasks to avoid one appearing or being more powerful than the other in the contribution made to the running of the group.
6. The use of themes and triggers that represent the experience of older people from the minority culture, in both their country of origin and adopted homeland.
7. Working out a mutually agreed strategy to counter any racist or prejudicial comments that arise in the group.

Factors that can act against a positive group reminiscence experience for members of a mixed cultural background include:

1. Group members from minority cultures finding it difficult to share with members from the white majority culture feelings and issues about any incidents of racism they have experienced.

2 Group members from the minority culture wanting or needing to communicate memories in their first language; interpretation into English may make the group process slow and cumbersome for all members.

3 The expression of strong racist or prejudicial views by group members.

PROMPTING MEMORIES IN GROUP AND ONE-TO-ONE REMINISCENCE WORK

Themes and triggers

When planning reminiscence group or one-to-one sessions it is important to identify appropriate triggers that will appeal to memories of life, both in the country of birth and the adopted homeland. Sources for culturally appropriate triggers may include older people; their family or friends; unit staff; libraries or museums; local places of worship.

The themes suggested in Chapter 4 are relevant when working with people from minority cultures. Also appropriate are the trigger suggestions which include artefacts, photographs, music, and quotes to prompt memories. Publications that include the memories of older people from minority cultures also provide excellent material for evocative quotes. A good source for such publications is Age Exchange, London. Two examples are *Remedies and Recipes – Caribbean Reflections on Health and Diet*, *A Place to Stay – Memories of Pensioners from Many Lands.*

Themes that involve a hands-on element are also excellent for stimulating memories in groups with mixed cultural membership. For example, preparing and eating traditional foods; showing others how traditional dress was, or is, worn; taking part in traditional craftwork.

THINKING POINT

Do you have experience of running reminiscence groups with a mixed cultural membership? Which themes were the most evocative for group members? Did these include any hands-on activities?

Themes related to celebrations

Prompting memories of religious and non-religious celebrations and festivals relating to a minority culture offers rich stimulus for recall, and often promotes lively discussion about how these events were observed in the past compared with the present day. In mixed membership groups, older people and leaders from different cultures can enjoy the 'living' history of another culture's rituals and celebrations.

Cultural identity can be maintained and valued by ensuring that important religious and non-religious celebrations are marked in settings where older people from minority cultures live or attend on a daily basis. Reminiscence groups can provide the focus for marking these special events with the preparation and eating of traditional foods, and music and dancing. In addition, it may be possible for older people to attend local community celebrations. For example, Chinese New Year celebrations take place in the Chinese Quarters of large cities; *Diwali*, a Hindu festival, is marked with light displays in the high streets of a number of towns and cities.

In the past, religious festivals and rituals played a large role in many older people's lives. Acknowledging, marking and celebrating these events in the present promotes continuity between the past and today; and observance of well-known and respected rituals increases a sense of security and familiarity. Some religious events demand the observance of rules about abstinence from food and drink. For example, throughout the month of Ramadan (dates change from year to year depending on the Islamic lunar calendar), Muslims are required to fast from dawn to sunset, in order to learn self-discipline and restraint. Older people are not required to fast, but memories of the impact of this observance in the past offer rich material for reminiscence work. Enjoyable memories could also be recalled about festivals such as *Id-ul-Fitr*, which takes place at the end of Ramadan, lasts three days and is often referred to as the 'Small Festival'.

Many older people take a great pride in their adherence to traditional religious practices in the past and present, and enjoy sharing memories that illustrate the strength of their faith. Traditional beliefs may have demanded the strict observance of the Sabbath (Saturday for followers of the Jewish faith, and Sunday for Christians), including worship in the local synagogue for people of the Jewish faith, or church for followers of the Christian faith. For followers of both faiths there would have been a belief in the need to refrain from all kinds of work on the Sabbath.

The sharing and comparing of experiences surrounding religious festivals and rituals offers rewarding possible outcomes for group members including the opportunity to increase understanding and knowledge of group members and leaders about the beliefs connected with another culture; reinforcement of cultural identity for group members; and the enlivening of everyday life through marking and celebrating festivals and other important cultural events.

Personal triggers

Reminiscence work on a one-to-one basis can be enriched by the use of triggers directly related to the interests, work or family life of individuals. Relevant triggers may belong to the individual (family photographs, music, books, postcards), or to family and friends. Alternatively, triggers that represent the life history and culture of the individual may be collected from outside sources.

Work on a one-to-one basis often focuses on the wish of the individual to produce a life-story or memories book, which records their life history. In this instance, the use of person- and culturally-specific triggers helps to promote and enrich the process of recall.

One-to-one work may also involve the expression of unresolved feelings of loss from the past, revived by bereavement or some other form of loss in the present, which may include moving into care. The opportunity to talk through feelings of loss with a listener who is culturally aware of the beliefs and rituals that hold meaning for the individual, offers a chance to share and express pain.

For further information on working with individuals see Chapter 7, 'Promoting One-to-One Reminiscence Work', which looks in detail at one-to-one work, including the role of bereavement and grieving in older people's lives and the preparation of life-story or memories books.

Summary Points

Reminiscence Across Cultures

- Sensitive and effective reminiscence work with people from minority cultures involves the acknowledgement, valuing and celebration of shared histories originating from diverse roots and experience.
- Awareness and understanding, on the part of reminiscence workers, about the impact of the experience of emigration on people from minority cultures increases sensitivity to the issues and accompanying feelings expressed during recall.
- Acknowledging the influence of cultural beliefs and attitudes on individuals, helps promote the personhood of caring regimes for people from minority cultures.
- Prompting inclusitivity within the reminiscence experience, for people from minority cultures, requires an awareness of issues to do with language barriers, co-working between leaders from the majority and minority cultures, transcultural group membership, and the use of culturally specific themes and triggers.
- Reminiscence work that focuses on marking and celebrating cultural festivals helps to maintain and transmit cultural heritage, while enriching everyday life for all.

7 Promoting One-to-One Reminiscence Work

Well everyone can master a grief but he that has it.
WILLIAM SHAKESPEARE, *Much Ado About Nothing*

This chapter focuses on how to promote reminiscence work on a one-to-one basis. The different forms that one-to-one reminiscence work can include are considered, together with the value that individual work plays in encouraging a personhood approach to the care of older people.

The time spent as a carer with older people on a one-to-one basis, using reminiscence work as a focus, provides a valuing way of celebrating the uniqueness of individuals who live in residential, day or community settings. The background information highlighted offers insights into the influences of the past on the make-up of individuals in the present. The personhood of older people is acknowledged and promoted by the interest shown in the fabric of individuals' past lives.

Different forms of one-to-one reminiscence work include:

- Promoting the recall of memories about various aspects of everyday life in the past related to individuals' family, home, school, neighbourhood, hobbies, interests and work, offers a valuing activity that maintains and builds self-esteem. Individuals may enjoy the opportunity to compile life-story or memories books as part of this one-to-one work.

- 'Being with' individuals as they 're-run' certain periods or events in their past lives that hold a strong negative or positive resonance. This 're-running' of the past may include a need to review roles played in life events, in order to come to terms with the past. This form of recall is referred to as 'life review work'.

- The opportunity for the repetition of bereavement reminiscences, which may include recalling the past relationship with the deceased, their personality, times shared, and details of the death and funeral. This repetition of recall plays a major role in the process of grieving; some bereaved individuals also find it helpful to prepare a life-story book, which provides an opportunity to record memories of the life shared with the deceased.

- Supporting individuals in their adjustment to the loss of home, mobility, hearing or sight.

- Identifying, based on information about the past, how the present can be enlivened with the renewal of former interests (possibly with modifications to allow for the changed circumstances of the individual).

The form of one-to-one reminiscence work undertaken with individuals varies; it may encompass one, several or all of the above areas. Work with each individual will be unique, depending on their situation, interests and needs.

LIFE HISTORY WORK

Older people involved in sharing aspects of their life history on a one-to-one basis with a carer, take part in a process that has the potential to increase self-awareness and esteem and enhance the relationship between carer and individual. Through telling their story, individuals are helped to mark and celebrate life events; re-evaluate difficult past experiences, recall special people and times, and generally sum up how their life map has worked out. A number of older people enjoy being helped to record details of their life history in the form of a life-story or memories book; others are content to recall their past without preserving a record.

The focus of life-history work may be to help an individual in the expression of bereavement reminiscences. In this instance, compiling a life-story book can be a way of acknowledging and preserving memories of the relationship with the deceased.

GETTING STARTED

Be clear with individuals about what a life-story or memories book is: how they are compiled; the kind of information that is usually included; the number of sessions needed to gather information; issues about confidentiality and ownership of the book.

Encourage the individual to make their own decision about involvement in life-story work. Emphasize that an unrecorded shared life history is just as valuable to the individual and listener as a recorded one.

Ensure sufficient time is available to prepare the life-story book; the overall time, and the length of individual sessions needed to gather personal information, varies depending on individual circumstances. For example, if an older person has dementia, sessions may need to be short but frequent. In total, the time required is unlikely to be less than three to four hours. Individual sessions of approximately one hour's duration work well. Additional time is required to collate the book and check out with the individual that they are in agreement with the content and presentation of the life-story record.

RECORDING A LIFE STORY

An individual may want to write down their own life story, with encouragement and help from the reminiscence worker. However, it is more common for older people to prefer the reminiscence worker to collate their recollections into a life-story book.

The worker may decide, with the individual's permission, to tape the interviews, and to transcribe the narrative later. This method has advantages in increasing accuracy and the ability to quote words and expressions used by individuals. In addition, for an older person with sight difficulties, an audio recording can form a valuable life-story 'talking' book.

The most common method used in recording memories for life-story books involves the worker taking notes during sessions, where possible recording the individual's exact words to personalise the subsequent life-story account. The disadvantages of this method of recording individuals' memories include the distraction element of note-taking, for both the individual and the listener. Non-verbal messages can be missed; individuals may speak quickly, reducing the accuracy of note-taking, or be stilted in their recall to enable the listener to 'get it all down'.

THINKING POINT

Think of an older person you hope to work with on their life-story book. Which method described do you think would be the most appropriate in recording memories during one-to-one sessions with the individual?

Content

It is important to appreciate that it is not possible to recall all aspects of an individual's life during life-story work: older people's past lives have spanned many years and been influenced by multiple personal and world events. However, reminiscence workers can gain and record a meaningful 'snapshot' of a life based on events that have been significant for an individual.

There are a number of pointers to think about when focusing on the content of life-story books:

What to include

Older people may not want everything shared with the reminiscence worker to be included in their life-story books. In the sessions, they express emotions about loss in their lives, including feelings of failure or guilt about certain situations. And they often express relief at having the opportunity to share feelings about past events. However, they do not usually wish this life-review work to be recorded.

Martha, who was in her nineties, wanted to compile a life-story book in order to leave behind a memory of herself for her children and grandchildren. But she was very clear that one painful episode in her life should not be recorded, as illustrated in the case study.

> During the one-to-one sessions, Martha happily recalled memories of her children when they were young; a number of stories recalled the pranks they got up to, and Martha was clear she wanted these recorded in her book, 'to make them laugh'. However, Martha's memories of her only son, Clive, in adulthood, were largely painful, due to the fact that she had disowned him for leaving his wife and children for another woman. Clive had only resumed contact with his mother a few years ago. Now Martha had an uneasy relationship with Clive, who still felt like 'a stranger' to her.
>
> Martha enjoyed recalling memories about Clive as a child, and looked relieved at having the opportunity to express long-held emotions about what she saw as the 'loss' of her son. However, she was very concerned to emphasize that recall about their long separation should not be referred to in her life-story book, as she did not want to upset Clive.

It is very important to check out with individuals what they wish to be included in their life account, both during individual sessions, and when the contents of the life-story book have been drafted.

Written and visual content

Individuals do not always recall memories in chronological order, and may have clearer memories about certain periods in their lives than others. Alternatively, recall may be more or less equal across the broad span of an older person's life. Generally, with age memories from the more distant past take on a sharper focus and are more to the forefront of the mind, making recall related to recent times less accessible. Although life-story books are generally collated in chronological order, it is not unusual to have unequal amounts of information about the different stages of an older person's life.

It is important that life-story accounts are written in the first person throughout, in order to promote personalisation of the contents, and to add to the sense of ownership experienced by individuals.

A life-story can be represented in many ways to bring alive the individuality of the content. An older person's background is powerfully illustrated by the inclusion of photographs of the subject and family members at different ages. Photographs of an individual's school, workplace or former home all add to the visual image of a life. Enlarged local maps, annotated to show where an individual was born, went to school and worked, can also be used to provide a visual representation of life.

Individuals may enjoy being asked to 'take a walk' down the street where they lived as a child, and recall the activity of the street, for example, neighbours; the milkman or other tradesmen who called; local shops; the route to school; street games. These recollections can be recorded in written form, or a simple drawing of the street can be made by the individual or the reminiscence worker, indicating the position of an individual's home, neighbours, shops, places of worship, or community halls. For older people from minority cultures, who immigrated to a new homeland, photographs and maps showing the country of origin are an excellent way of valuing and celebrating an individual's life.

Postcards or photographs of favourite holidays can be included. Individuals may have retained tickets or programmes relating to shows, concerts or sports matches they have attended; and the inclusion of these and similar items says a great deal about individuals' past interests.

Words can be used in various forms to represent an older person's story. They may have a favourite poem they wish to be included; the individual or someone they have been close to may have written poetry or short stories, and one or more of these could be 'published' in the life-story book. A saying or sayings that sum up an individual's philosophy towards life could also be recorded.

A person's background can also be represented by the inclusion of photographs illustrating a job of work undertaken by the individual or a relative. In the same way, illustrations or photographs of a favourite pastime can also be included. (See Katie's case study.)

Katie's father had been a blacksmith in their village. She did not have any photographs of him at work, but was pleased to include in her life-story book a general illustration of a blacksmith at his forge. One of Katie's interests, and a source of income for her family, had been knitting; to represent this interest she chose to include an old pattern for knitting a woollen suit, similar to the one she recalled knitting for five shillings for a friend. Katie enjoyed holding and examining five shillings in 'old' money, and marvelling at how little it was possible to buy today for the equivalent in 'new' money.

The personalised triggers relating to Katie's past added to the enjoyment of her memories, and their appeal to both her sense of seeing and touch gave added stimulus to her recall. The photograph and objects from the past provided a visual representation of important elements in her life-story.

Promoting recall

Individuals vary in the kind of prompts that facilitate recall of memories. Some need only the focus of one question about their past to spark off a chain of recollections; for others, part of each session may be dominated by the repetition of one or more favourite or difficult memories.

For many older people prompts using personal triggers help to bring the past to life. Family photographs, pictures, paintings, even items of furniture, all offer possibilities for use as effective triggers to recall. Existing knowledge about an older person may also suggest appropriate triggers that the worker can use in sessions to stimulate recall. Triggers that hold both personal relevance and sensory appeal have particular potential for evoking the recall of past memories, as illustrated in this case study.

In his first life-story book session, John had talked about his grandmother, who had played a domineering matriarchal role in his family. One of John's enduring memories of his grandmother centred on the smell of mothballs, which always lingered on her clothes. In the following session, John's reminiscence worker took with her a box of mothballs to act as a trigger to prompt memories of John's grandmother. As soon as the worker entered his room, John laughed in recognition of the strong smell and was soon talking avidly about past memories of his grandmother.

John's personal trigger in this life-story session was a particularly potent one, evoking humour and enjoyable recall.

A well-remembered piece of music, or a favourite song, often acts as an evocative trigger in life-story work, transporting individuals back to the past and prompting recall of events.

THINKING POINT

Think about a favourite song from your own past. If it is available, listen to it again. What effect does it have on you? Are you transported back to another time, and reminded of events associated with the era of the song?

Returning to local areas where older people lived as children and adults can be effective in stimulating recollections of the past. Photographs taken on these visits to well-remembered places can enliven life-story books. There may be particular landmarks that individuals wish to visit: some will be largely unchanged by the passage of time; others will have altered, possibly beyond recognition. It is important that individuals are aware of what to expect before returning to once-familiar neighbourhoods.

Using this method of revisiting neighbourhoods in order to stimulate recall in life-story work needs handling very sensitively. A number of older people will prefer to remember significant places as they were in the past, and not as they are in the present. Additionally, former neighbourhoods can hold many memories associated with loss. In particular, seeing again the home lived in immediately before moving to residential care can provoke distress.

Visiting local heritage museums may hold interest for individuals in relation to former occupations or hobbies, and may offer excellent prompts to recall. Additionally, past interests and skills may be revitalised through these visits, which also provide an excellent opportunity for collecting information to include in the individual's life-story book.

Some older people may enjoy being shown how to obtain information via the internet and the world-wide web, about, for example, past interests, occupations and local or far-away places they have had connections with. Information gained in this way affords stimulus to recall; links the past powerfully with the present, and provides the chance for older people to participate in a contemporary technology.

With the growing use of laptop computers, the internet is becoming increasingly accessible for use in community and residential settings. Where the expertise and/or equipment is not available within care settings, it may be possible to forge links with local schools or other community groups who would be interested in showing older people and their carers how to use the internet and world-wide web resources. As a result of sharing their expertise in this way, volunteers are in turn introduced to the fund of memories and knowledge that older people possess, and that could provide a valuable resource for the wider community.

Confidentiality and ownership

In terms of confidentiality, an older person sharing emotions about life review situations needs to feel secure that a life-story book, or any other form of life-story record, is confidential, with the individual having full control over both content and who sees the record. Additionally, it is important to stress that any taped or written record of an older person's life is their property and does not belong to the reminiscence worker or the care setting.

A further ownership issue in life-story work is to find out what individuals wish to happen to the record of their life when they die. Life-story work often prompts thoughts about death and discussion of the older person's beliefs, or the lack of them, and about what happens after death. This kind of discussion often provides a good opening to talk with the individual about who they wish to own their life-story record after their death. The choice for some older people about ownership of their story after death is easier than for others, as illustrated by Elizabeth's case study.

Elizabeth had enjoyed being helped to compile her life-story book, and on its completion was looking forward to showing it to each of her four children. When asked which of her children she wanted to have the book after her death, she smiled and without hesitation replied, 'Oh, the one who shows the most enjoyment and interest in it, of course!'

For many older people, choices in terms of who may like the record of their life are often more limited and less clear-cut than for Elizabeth; and feelings of sadness may be evoked by a lack of any remaining sense of belonging to others. However, in instances where an older person has no surviving friends or relatives, it may be possible to identify a carer who the individual feels close to, and whom they would wish to have their life-story. Alternatively, the reminiscence worker may be able to reassure the older person that they would like the book as a permanent reminder of them.

Past, present and future

It is essential not to view life-story books as being complete at any given point: individuals' life stories go on; and older people need to feel valued for who they are in the past, present and future. A life-story book provides a tool for tracking and recording happenings in older people's past *and* present lives. Photographs of individuals taking part in activities, including local trips out or celebrations within the care setting, can be included. Important events within individuals' families can also be recorded, such as anniversaries or births.

By including references to the past and the present, older people are helped to maintain a sense of the past linking with and flowing into the present and the future. Through the recording process, individuals' lives are valued and given continuity. Additionally, for carers, the life-story record provides an ongoing and meaningful prompt to facilitate regular discussion about events, places and interests, past and present, that have shaped an individual's world.

LIFE-STORY WORK AND PEOPLE WITH DEMENTIA

The initial reaction of carers when considering life-story work, with people with dementia, tends to be that the process appears very difficult to undertake, due to the often splintered and elusive nature of individuals' memories. John Killick, a writer-in-residence in care settings for older people, illustrates how it is possible and valuable to help people with dementia record their feelings and views on past and present life, however fragmented their recall. Killick (1994) describes how, by acting initially as an amanuensis (a person who writes to dictation), he takes down thoughts expressed by individuals about their life, which often contain symbolism, and arranges them into personalised poetic format. This poetry acts as a form of life-story work, and is subsequently shared, where appropriate, with the individual, staff, and relatives.

Through this kind of work, insights may be provided for carers into individuals' feelings about their present situation, and these can make a valuable contribution to the formulation of effective care plans. Additionally, individuals feel they are being heard and valued in their recall of the past: Edie, who with John Killick's help wrote a poem called *Wandering*, sums up the value of sharing her current life experience in the last verse of the poem:

> That's a nice little piece
> of writing you've done. It's better
> that, love, than nothing.
> I hope it does something for you.
> My memory, it slims away...

To fail to engage people with dementia in life-story work, in whatever form, is to deny them an opportunity to celebrate their unique life history. Life-story work with people with dementia can play a key role in promoting and strengthening the personhood of individuals. Taking part in this kind of reminiscence work highlights to carers and older people the intricate patterns of past lives, and the individuality still to be communicated through recall.

The focus of life-story work with people with dementia offers a valuable contribution to the quality of individuals' social and emotional wellbeing by:

- Reducing the fragmenting effects of dementia on social relationships between individuals and their carers: knowledge about individuals' lives can provide highly personalised and relevant topics of conversation.
- Illuminating the rich diversity of individuals' lives, which helps to illustrate the uniqueness of all older people, and promotes heightened awareness in carers of the variation in the life maps followed by individuals.
- Returning shared memories subsequently lost with the inexorable advance of dementia, and maintaining an individual's sense of self for a longer period.
- Affording empathetic, one-to-one attention to individuals, who are thus helped to sense their place in the past and present world. The uniqueness of personal experience is marked and celebrated, in part by the interest and understanding shown by the reminiscence worker.
- Gaining background history about older people with dementia which, however fragmented, provides meaningful and insightful glimpses into the make-up of individuals.
- 'Tuning in' to verbal and non-verbal clues provided by people with dementia, which facilitates understanding of the feelings and emphasis that is being communicated about the past and present, through what may initially appear to be disjointed and difficult to understand recall.
- Appreciating that valuable indicators as to who were past significant figures in individuals' lives are communicated through poignant and often repetitive requests relating, for example, to seeing deceased parents and spouses.
- Extending background knowledge about individuals, which helps to ease times when pain about the past and present becomes overwhelming. Empathetically, individuals can be helped through the positive diversion of renewing enriching links with the past (see also Chapter 5, 'Reminiscence Work and the Challenge of Dementia').
- Reconnecting individuals, in some form, with past interests highlighted through the life-story work process, and so giving pleasure-in-the-moment.

Promoting recall

When working with people with dementia on their life-story account, reminiscence workers need as much background information as possible about individuals. Where memory even about the distant past is decreasing, and/or lacking in continuity, the more specific and personally relevant triggers to memory need to be in order to evoke recall. To supplement the information available from individuals with dementia, relatives, friends, staff and existing files may be able to provide additional background. Relatives or friends can be helped to recall information about the individual by using the Group Member's Profile Form (see Chapter 3, 'Reminiscence Groups – The Planning Stage').

Personal photographs or other items may be available to trigger memories. When using photographs, the worker should ideally be aware of the names of individuals in the photographs, their relationship to the person with dementia, and details of any past or present sensitive issues arising from the relationship. This kind of background knowledge considerably enhances the effectiveness of photographs as triggers to recall.

References made earlier in this chapter to the evocative power of sensory triggers also apply when working with people with dementia, particularly where triggers relate to specific personal experience and preferences.

Background information obtained through reminiscence 'research' with Arthur, a widower in his eighties who was experiencing dementia, and his family showed that music would be a valuable personal trigger to use in work with Arthur.

Playing a cello had been very important to Arthur in his youth. He had also enjoyed listening to cello music, and had once heard Jacqueline Dupree in concert playing Elgar's *Cello Concerto*. On hearing a CD of the same concerto, Arthur became lost in the music and suddenly, with a twinkle in his eye, mimed picking up a cello and playing the instrument.

For Arthur, the sensory effect of a specific piece of well-known and loved music had evoked memories of an accomplishment he had been very proud of in his youth. It had created pleasure-in-the-moment for him, providing an opportunity to acknowledge and help maintain part of his unique personhood. For the reminiscence worker, this was a very moving and enjoyable moment to share with Arthur. It also strongly illustrated the power of specific reminiscence cues to link the past with the present in an enriching bond.

Arthur's family were moved to hear of his continuing love of the cello, and the concerto was subsequently played at his funeral, thus acknowledging and celebrating one of Arthur's many interests and achievements.

In this instance, reminiscence work can be clearly seen to link not only, the past with the present, but additionally the past and present with the future. For Arthur's family and friends, this piece of music is likely to remain associated with memories of him in the future. In this way reminiscence can weave memory threads through time.

THINKING POINT

Could you help an individual you care for to rediscover a piece of music, or a song that once gave them pleasure, and find out if the music relates to a meaningful memory?

Some older people with dementia retain a clear and detailed 'window' of memory around a particular period in their life. Initial life-story work sessions may highlight a time or event to which an individual repeatedly returns to in their recall. If this is the case, it is valuable and enjoyable for individuals if the reminiscence worker focuses life-story work on their particular 'window' of memory. Having a selective, but restricted, focus for life-story work may also be necessary if personal information is limited about an individual's general background.

Felicity, who experienced dementia, had lived in a nursing home for three years. There was little background information available about her life, as her husband and other relatives had died. However, once Felicity had revealed a 'window' of retained memory, life-story work proved very enjoyable to her.

Felicity regularly attended group reminiscence, and one day a reference to pocket money triggered for her many memories of a happy childhood in Scotland. Throughout the session, Felicity talked about aspects of her early life in the Scottish borders, showing a very unusual animation.

Felicity was subsequently involved in life-story work sessions during which her retained 'window' of long-term memory focused sharply on pleasurable recall about her father's work as a farmer and her early years at school. Recall was prompted by the use of triggers, including pictures of farmers at work and Magnolia trees, which had been Felicity's favourite tree in her childhood garden.

Focusing Felicity's life-story book on this small, but important, part of her life gave her great pleasure in the initial recall, and ongoing enjoyment whenever she was shown her book. Felicity would often say with a smile, when looking at her book, 'See, I can remember all that', showing evident pleasure that one part of her memory was still intact.

Felicity's carers were shown a previously unknown part of her life through her life-story book. Before this, it had been difficult for carers to refer to Felicity's past, due to her decreasing memory and their lack of background history. However, Felicity's key worker now felt a greater confidence in talking to her about the past; the life-story book provided a focus for enjoyable and mutually rewarding discussions.

THINKING POINT

Do you care for a person with dementia for whom you have little background information, but who regularly talks about one period or event in their life? How could you increase your background knowledge prior to undertaking one-to-one life-story work with that person?

FORMAT OF LIFE-STORY PRESENTATION

Many older people enjoy having a written record of their life in the form of a life-story book, but this kind of record is not everyone's preference. It is useful to have a repertoire of ideas about how recall in life-story work can be recorded and preserved. The following is a selection of different kinds of life-story records:

1 Life-story books include a written and visual record of an individual's life. Information can be displayed in loose-leaf files, which facilitate easy movement and addition of information. Alternatively, books can be used with a specifically designed format for recording life-story work.

2 Photo albums can be compiled of snapshots of relatives and friends, and favourite places. Including a record of names and relationships increases the effectiveness of the album as a trigger for recall.

3 Large photo-boards or frames can be put in individuals' rooms, displaying personal photographs of past significant people and places. An advantage of this kind of record is that the photo-board or frame forms a prominent feature acting as an effective instant visual stimulus to individuals, and a talking point for visitors. Additionally, the contents of the photo-board or frame can be changed easily to keep the interest and attention of the individual and their carers.

4 A sound-recording on audiotape of an individual recalling their life offers a highly personalised record that captures the person's characteristic intonations of voice. For individuals with sight difficulties a sound recording has obvious benefits in supplementing or replacing the written word when recording a life-history record.

5 A video record can be made of individuals talking about their lives. However, to make this an accessible method of recording life history, that avoids too much repetition, time-consuming, skilled editing is essential. But a short video recording could be valuable in supplementing a life-story book, bringing 'life' into the written record.

6 Family trees can be drawn up to represent individuals' past ancestry and present family. Computer packages are available to help formulate family trees and more extensive life history records. (For example, *The Family Tree Maker* produced by Broderbund.)

7 Memory books can be compiled, based solely on individuals' major interests or hobbies. Past and present-day material about an interest can be included. An example of this style of life-history record is an individual who had been a member of a cycling club: photographs of days out with the club; maps of routes followed; local newspaper cuttings about club activities; history of the club, or cycling generally, could all be incorporated in their book.

In the USA, there is a growing interest in promoting the writing and preservation of life-story work through 'guided autobiography'. John Kunz (1999) discusses the work of Thelma Kramer, an important proponent of this method of life-story work. Guided autobiography involves older people being encouraged, sometimes in a community group setting, to write and read out loud, stories from their life. Kramer believes that guided autobiography has a major role to play in increasing the self-esteem of older people through the celebration of their lives.

Kramer describes 'the lift' experienced by senior adults in telling their story on stage in front of other older people. One guided autobiography course run by Kramer was called 'Life Tapestries'. Kramer compared the intricacy of the stories created on the course to verbal tapestries:

> We adopted the name, Life Tapestries, because the stories we were weaving with words were so unique that each one became a verbal tapestry.

Many stories written by senior adults are subsequently published in the magazine *One of a Kind: The Caregiver's Voice*, which is edited by Thelma Kramer.

Life-story work, in whatever form, provides opportunities in residential, day-care settings and individuals' own homes for enhancing relationships between carers and older people: holding the power to illuminate the past history of individuals while breathing new life and interest into the present.

LIFE-STORY WORK AND THE FUTURE

With dramatically increasing numbers of older people who are unable to live alone, as a result of mental and/or physical health difficulties, cost and good practice implications are forcing governments in Europe and the USA to look at alternatives to permanent residential care for individuals. Life-story work has a meaningful role to play in the future, in the care of older people both in and outside residential units. Its ability to provide an insightful and meaningful link with the past, in the present, provides a potential focus for social interaction where community or day-centre teams of carers are involved in maintaining older people in their own homes.

One-to-one reminiscence work has the potential to help carers build initial and ongoing relationships with older people in innovative care schemes, such as the US project known as 'senior fostering'. James Bennett (2000), reporting on this scheme, describes it as one that matches older people with couples or families who are able to offer care in their own home, for which they receive training and a weekly payment.

For older people with very high dependency care needs, due to mental health difficulties, there is a growing view that supports the future use of small-scale residential and day-care units that are able to recreate domestic-style living environments for people with dementia. Again, in this kind of care setting, life-story work offers an invaluable way of personalising the care relationship, by illustrating the uniqueness of all individuals.

BEREAVEMENT AND OLDER PEOPLE

Frequently, one-to-one reminiscence work involves understanding and responding to older people's reactions to complex loss histories. The remainder of this chapter therefore provides information about: the kinds of losses experienced by older people; phases and tasks of grieving; empathetic responses to loss reactions; the role of bereavement reminiscence, and complicated grieving reactions. Developing insight into the role played by bereavement in one-to-one reminiscence work helps carers to respond sensitively to older people when their recall is associated with loss.

EXPERIENCES OF LOSS

Bereavement is normally associated with the death of someone significant in an individual's life. Although the death of a loved one is the most severe loss that can be experienced, it is essential to appreciate that loss reactions in older people can also be provoked by the absence of *something*, as well as someone, that is significant and precious in their lives. Feelings of loss may be experienced about a former home, or be provoked by a more general loss, such as independence. Initial, and ongoing bereavement reactions can arise from any loss that is perceived as significant by an individual.

Discernible feelings of loss expressed in bereavement reminiscences may centre on multiple deaths experienced by the older person in their past and present life. Additionally, painful memories associated with the death of loved ones in the past may be heightened by new experiences of significant loss, such as that of a familiar way of life following admission to residential care.

THINKING POINT

Think of an older person you have previously or are currently caring for. What major losses connected with the past are you aware they have experienced? Are there also present losses related to changes in their way of life that they refer to?

The possible losses that older people may wish or need to focus on in life-history work are myriad:

- Older people may not have known their natural parents as a result of being fostered or adopted as babies. Knowledge about natural parents may have been gained late in life, and some older people will have had to grieve the death of both birth and adopted parents.

- Siblings may have died as children or adults. These deaths may have been in sudden and tragic circumstances.

- Individuals may have grown old in an adopted homeland: life as a member of a minority culture within any society has the potential to create many loss experiences.

- Long-term relationships in adulthood may have ended as a result of death, divorce or separation. Major changes in lifestyle may have resulted from broken relationships: unemployment, poverty, house moves, loss of status and support generally.

- Individuals may have experienced infertility possibly leading to childlessness. Alternatively, babies may have died due to miscarriage or stillbirth.

- Children may have died before reaching adulthood or during adulthood. This is a particularly common experience for older women who often outlive their sons. Statistics from the USA, published by the Metropolitan Life Insurance Company (1977), showed that women aged over 65 with a living son had a one in four chance of surviving their child. Parents do not expect to outlive their children, and the death of a child, whatever their age, can be particularly traumatic.

- Personal ambitions and happiness may have been thwarted, due to limiting traditional gender roles or problematic relationships.

- Death of parents is a very painful loss for most people, but grief reactions may be heightened in intensity and duration if older people did not leave the parental home to live independently in adulthood.

- Loss of autonomy may have resulted from problems with physical or mental health.

- A move to a residential care setting results in the loss of home; many possessions; pets, and familiar routines. Choices may be more restrictive; there is the need to adapt to living in a large setting with others, perhaps for the first time in an individual's life. The move to residential care is one of the most demanding changes faced by an older person. A change that has to be contended with at a time when an individual may be physically and mentally at their most vulnerable.

COPING WITH GRIEF

One factor viewed by many gerontologists as strongly influencing how older people cope with bereavement and loss is the disenfranchising (undervaluing) of their grief by the rest of society. This involves at worst the negation and, at best, the minimisation of the extent of older people's feelings towards personal loss. Two American researchers, Miriam and Sydney Moss (1996), consider that the isolation and feelings of disconnection from others, common following bereavement, are compounded by the lack of acknowledgement of the depth of older people's grief. In instances such as the death of an adult son or daughter, primary attention and care is often directed towards the spouse and children of the deceased, not the surviving parent.

Doka (1989) considers that older people experience a disenfranchisement of their grief when the impact of personal loss is undervalued, resulting in an absence, or inadequacy of bereavement support, from formal and informal support systems. Reminiscence work provides a valuable support system for bereaved older people. One-to-one work with individuals that focuses sensitively on bereavement reminiscences provides an effective way to acknowledge and value older people's grief.

EMPATHETIC WAYS OF RESPONDING TO BEREAVEMENT REMINISCENCES

- Acknowledging the extent of pain felt, and the value of the relationship or significant *something* that has been lost.
- Being able to recognise when loss in the present results in the need for individuals to revisit loss episodes from the past.
- Offering explanations and reassurance about normal feelings and reactions experienced following bereavement.
- If an individual is from a minority culture, ensuring sufficient is known about personal beliefs and traditions associated with death and grieving in order to offer culturally appropriate support to the older person.
- Initiating the recording of memories, where appropriate, to enable an individual to preserve recall about the deceased and their shared life.
- Identifying interests and activities that retain the ability to provide pleasure-in-the-moment for individuals, to help them attain some momentary respite from feelings of loss.

All the above empathetic responses value individuals' experiences of grief, and ensure that older people are respected and treated as unique individuals. Individualising responses made to older people who have been bereaved offers a positive counter to the well-meaning but minimising sympathy expressed through platitudes, such as 'Don't be sad, she had a good innings', or over-reassurance that denies the pain of loss, 'You will feel better soon, time is a great healer.' Scrutton (1995) considers that reassurance made up of bland, empty responses is a devaluing reaction to the emotional upheaval being experienced by bereaved older people:

> Bereaved people can be reassured that they are not alone or unsupported but they cannot be reassured that they have not suffered loss.

Platitudes relating to experiences surrounding death do not all deny the reality of loss, and may even be used by older people themselves to express their feelings about bereavement. However, the inappropriate use of platitudes can result in a minimisation of older people's reaction to loss, or have the effect of blocking the expression of normal distress. This is particularly so in instances where the message communicated by the platitude is not congruent with an individual's current phase of grieving. An example would be quoting platitudes that emphasize recovery from loss in the early phase of bereavement: 'Life must go on' and 'Time is a great healer'. At this point, individuals naturally need to focus on the shock of loss, and may feel guilty and disloyal even contemplating a time when they will be over their loss.

The effect of loss on older people is often minimised due to the expectation that familiarity with death, through past losses, shields older people against the painful onslaught of grief. This view denies both the individuality of each loss experience, and the potential power of sequential significant losses to cause emotional overload, depriving some older people of the resources to cope with repeated grief. For some individuals, this emotional overload can be provoked by simultaneously trying to come to terms with a resurgence of pain from the past and loss of significant people and/or familiar patterns of living in the present.

An additional loss area for older people living in communal residential settings is the death of fellow residents. Carers may undervalue the impact of this loss. For some older people these deaths act as a powerful emotional reminder of the proximity of their own mortality, together with feelings of loss for newly formed friendships. In this situation, older people may be hurt about how quickly all memory of the deceased resident's presence is removed from the home, and someone else unceremoniously supplanted in their room.

Carers, witnessing how older people sometimes seem to be surrounded by death and other significant loss, can feel a natural desire to reduce the effects of this continual emotional bombardment from loss. So they feel it is best to avoid all reference to deceased relatives or friends. However, the experience of loss does not go away if ignored, and sometimes avoidance of the subject is about self-protection on the carer's part: personal coping strategies when faced with death may be to move on and not think about loss. Focusing on another's grief may provoke fears about a carer's own death, or the death of significant people in their own life.

Desiring to protect others from emotional pain is understandable, but may result in avoidance or difficulty, on the carer's part, in 'being with' older people as they experience natural and healing grief about loss situations. Valuable opportunities may be missed to: affirm older people's bereavement feelings and reactions; allay fears; hear, acknowledge and celebrate the memories of an individual, or way of life, now lost to the older person. Acknowledging personal reactions to loss, and seeking support in sharing pain about actual or feared losses, helps carers to remove or reduce the blocks constructed by personal fears, which hinder the capacity to sensitively 'be with' older people in bereavement situations.

PHASES AND TASKS OF GRIEVING

The process of grieving is referred to variously as passing through 'stages' or 'phases'; accomplishing 'tasks', or facing the 'conflicts' of grief. Despite the different terminology adopted in describing the grieving process, there is general agreement between writers and researchers working in this field, that the process is a long one, with an emotional ebb and flow of feelings to be faced.

Individuals do not follow an ordered chronological path through the psychological process of grieving and there is no set time for the completion of grieving. Individuals often experience one set of emotions and reactions only for them to return later in the grieving process. For example, the raw feelings of missing the deceased person associated with the period immediately following death may recur a year later around the anniversary of the death. Lewis (1966) succinctly describes this confusing but normal process of emerging from and returning to the different phases of grief following the death of his wife:

> One keeps on emerging from a phase, but it always recurs. Round and round. Everything repeats. Am I going in circles, or dare I hope I am on a spiral? But if a spiral, am I going up or down it?

Certain reactions and feelings appear common to individuals following a loss but everyone is different. Many factors in an older person's life, including personality; previous experiences; resolution of past losses; present sequential losses; support systems and religious beliefs, all affect how individuals cope with the grieving process.

An appreciation of the role of diverse cultural and religious beliefs associated with death and dying is essential. Many older people gain comfort from a strong religious faith at times of loss, and will be helped if they are enabled to follow religious rituals and grieving traditions.

Being aware of the feelings and reactions associated with coping with loss helps carers to listen and respond to bereavement reminiscences with informed sensitivity and empathy. For example, knowing that repetitive recall about a deceased individual, or a lost way of life, is part of the process of coming to terms with loss may help carers to respond with ongoing empathy. It is essential, too, to avoid imposing an anticipated formula or time-scale to older people's grieving patterns: the complexity of individuals and their experience needs to be responded to in a way that acknowledges their uniqueness.

Reminiscence workers may be challenged with helping older people to cope with the phases and accompanying tasks of grieving at different points in their work with individuals. Significant people may die during the older person's involvement in life-history work, resulting in the recall of past losses being stimulated by the pain of present loss. Alternatively, loss of a way of life, due to increasing physical and/or mental health difficulties, may prompt bereavement reminiscences about more independent times.

A general guide to the kinds of feelings and reactions experienced by bereaved people, is given by Leick and Davidsen-Nielsen (1991), who describe the four tasks that individuals facing loss have to accomplish:

1. Accepting the reality of loss

2. Entering into the emotions and dealing with resultant feelings

3. Acquisition of new skills for a future without the deceased

4. Reinvestment of energy in order to form new relationships

Leick and Davidsen-Nielsen, writing without specific consideration of older people's experience of loss, believe that these four tasks overlap and intermingle from the time of loss, and need to be worked on, at different times and with varying intensity, throughout the duration of grieving.

This section includes a detailed look at the phases and tasks of grieving experienced by individuals after a bereavement involving the loss of someone or *something* significant in their lives. Information is included that gives pointers on how to respond to typical comments made, and reactions experienced by older people during different phases of the grieving process.

INITIAL PHASE: ABSORBING THE REALITY OF THE LOSS EVENT

The first phase of grieving involves achieving the task of realisation, on an emotional as well as a practical reasoning level, that a loss has taken place. During this initial phase, the loss can be such a major shock that the mind initially resists experiencing fully the devastating pain of separation. This protective resistance may take the form of numbness, which many people describe as feeling disconnected from reality in the period immediately following a death. A sense of 'going through the motions', without really feeling involved, is often experienced. Individuals who experience this reaction of numbness may later find it difficult to fully recall the immediate events following a major loss.

Freda Baker (1992), writing about the initial period following the death of her husband, succinctly describes the feeling of numbness often experienced at this time:

> I was living in a no-man's-land, where there is no day or night, no yesterday, today or tomorrow.

For some individuals, this initial phase may involve fluctuating between the disconnected sensation of being removed or at a distance from events, and feeling keenly part of what is happening, responding to those around and taking part in any planning and decision-making required.

Denial of a death can also be a normal early response to grief: the mind cannot tolerate, even temporarily, the awareness of loss. Denial offers a 'breathing space' before having to register the severity of the loss and cope with its implications for the future. The more sudden, untimely, tragic or significant the loss, the more likely it is to provoke a reaction of initial denial. However extreme this response to the obvious fact of death appears to carers, it is important to be aware that, for some individuals, denial is an early normal reaction to major loss.

Searching for the lost individual is another normal coping technique that may surface in the early days of grief and, on occasions, during later phases of grieving. Searching enables the bereaved individual to delay accepting final separation from the deceased; searching may not necessarily be all-consuming, but involves an intermittent overwhelming desire for reconnection with the deceased. Common searching responses include continuing to lay the table with a place for the deceased; listening for and 'hearing' familiar noises previously connected with the deceased; 'seeing' the individual in familiar places in the home, and 'seeing' people in the street who resemble the deceased and believing momentarily it is them.

These instances of searching, however transitory, can be powerful experiences for bereaved individuals, and can be experienced as frustrating, upsetting and unsettling incidents. Equally, some individuals gain momentary relief from their loss, and may view these searching experiences as proof that the deceased is still with them in some way.

Slowly, as individuals begin to absorb the reality of loss, even from an initial position of denial, painful emotions, often accompanied by tears, begin to surface as they face the impact of death.

THINKING POINT

Are you currently aware of an older person who has recently experienced bereavement? If so do you recognise, in their responses, any of the reactions or feelings described in the first phase of grieving?

Responding to bereavement reactions in the initial phase

- Acknowledgement of the momentousness of the loss experienced, and reassurance of how difficult it can be initially to assimilate the reality and meaning of a death, is valuable when older people express concern about feelings of numbness:

> 'Your sister was such a daily support to you, it is not surprising that you find it difficult to believe she is dead; it is usual for a loss like this to take a while to sink in.'

- Avoid reinforcing any denial by gently referring to the person who has died, the relationship to the bereaved, and acknowledging the significance of the loss. An empathetic response to an older person whose son has just died would be:

> 'What a shock you have had, Brian's death was so unexpected. Often a major loss like yours is very hard to take in at first, how are you managing?'

- Where the bereaved older person is distressed about their searching response to a death, it is important to stress the normality of this reaction, and offer reassurance that it does not indicate mental health problems:

> 'Brian's death has been a major sudden loss, it will take time for you to absorb what has happened. It is common for people to think they 'see' the person who has died in a public or familiar place. Some people find comfort in this kind of experience, but others feel upset by it.'

SECOND PHASE: FACING THE EMOTIONAL PAIN OF LOSS

This second phase of grieving can be lengthy and very painful. At this time, it is very important for reminiscence workers to 'be with' older people, listening and responding with words and touch, when appropriate, to bereavement reminiscences associated with the deceased.

Individuals move into this phase of grieving as the reality of the loss is slowly absorbed. One of the tasks associated with this phase is to experience the painful emotions and reactions to loss that regularly overwhelm people who have been bereaved. Tears often accompany distress and despair about the loss, and profound missing of the deceased. Bereavement reminiscences at this time are likely to be numerous, possibly repetitious, and include many memories of the deceased, covering all aspects of their life.

There may be a need through bereavement reminiscences to 'sort out' the details of a death. This is a particularly common response when death happens in tragic circumstances, or out of the natural order of life. The process of attempting to understand why and how a loss happened is undertaken to make sense of the experience, and often involves determining if everything possible was done to prevent the death.

The attempt often made in this phase to 'sort out' why and how a significant loss took place can also be observed in older people's bereavement reminiscences, relating to changes in their living situations. Bereavement reminiscences focusing on an older person's last home can be especially poignant and persistent. A particularly difficult experience for individuals is moving to a residential setting straight from hospital, without the opportunity to visit their home for the last time. Strong feelings of loss are often experienced, and there is a need to try to make sense of why life has suddenly been turned upside down.

THINKING POINT

Can you think of an older person you care for who expresses bereavement reminiscences about their former home and shows distress at the loss? Did they have the opportunity to say goodbye to their home?

Anger and guilt reactions

In this phase of grieving, individuals may experience emotions of anger and guilt. These uncomfortable emotions may be directed at self, others or the deceased. Blame may be apportioned if the bereaved feels that not enough was done to prevent the death, and anger may be directed at the deceased for leaving the individual to cope alone with so much. The latter expressions of anger are often quickly followed by guilt at being so selfish and uncaring about the deceased. Guilt and anger are particularly common emotions expressed in circumstances where a loss is untimely, sudden or tragic. For example, an older person whose adult child has died often expresses guilt at having survived their offspring, feeling strongly that they should have died first.

All these emotions and reactions are normal within the grieving process, and although painful to express are part of the process of reconciling individuals to their loss.

Task of healing

This phase of grief is about promoting the task of healing following a major loss, through an often drawn out period of facing the emotions of loss; recalling memories of the deceased, and going over and over the details of the circumstances of loss. Distressing emotions and poignant memories cannot be endured unceasingly, and a healthy, normal response to this phase of grieving is to move in and out of a confrontation with the pain of loss.

The open wound of grief begins to heal slowly during this phase. Individuals, although still missing the deceased, experience the emotions of grief more intermittently, and often with less intensity. There is a growing, if fluctuating, feeling of having faced, and survived the depths of grief. The deceased has not been 'left behind' by the bereaved individual, on the contrary, the process of facing the emotions of loss and experiencing the recall of bereavement reminiscences may, for some, create a feeling that the deceased has been integrated to a lesser or greater extent into their way of being. This feeling of integration with the deceased is experienced as a positive support for coping in the future.

During this phase of grieving, it will be necessary for individuals to face alone important events that were previously shared including birthdays, wedding anniversaries, Christmas and other traditional celebrations. In addition, at the end of the first year, the anniversary of the death has to be faced. This event may, temporarily, cause the bereaved to experience some or all of the earlier emotions and reactions to loss, albeit with less intensity and duration.

Responding to bereavement reactions in the second phase

- Being empathetically responsive to bereavement reminiscences about the deceased, however repetitive, is an invaluable way of helping older people cope with this phase of grieving:

  'George, you have shared so many special memories with me about your life with Mabel together with thoughts about how her death happened. This kind of remembering is very important in helping you feel easier, over time, about Mabel's death.'

- Offering reassurance about the normality of the extent and kind of emotions individuals are experiencing is important. When a spouse has died, and grief seems long-lived to the individual, it can be helpful to point out that relationships of long duration and deep meaning cannot be recovered from in a short time and without pain:

  'Six months must seem a long time to be feeling so low about Mabel's death, George, but you were together many, many years. Your feelings of continuing loss show how much you cared for Mabel and miss her now.'

- Coupled with reassurance about the normality of duration and intensity of feelings experienced in bereavement, it is important to talk about how healing in loss takes place, and about how there will be a time when grief will be less overwhelming:

  'All the pain you feel at the moment, George, is upsetting, but slowly you will begin to feel easier, and be able to think of Mabel and her death without always being overcome with such distress and loss.'

- Older people may be embarrassed and overwhelmed by the expression of emotions related to their loss. It is essential that they feel accepted and not judged in sharing painful emotions. Being empathetically alongside individuals in the healing of grief through their release of emotions and tears is an invaluable response. At times of deep distress, a shared hug can offer unspoken acceptance and caring:

  'You look close to tears, George, you may feel easier if you allow them to come. Tears can help release some of your pain.'

- As the first anniversary of the death approaches, it is valuable to 'sound out' how the older person views this, and if they have plans about how to spend the day. Explanations and reassurance about the normality of experiencing the anniversary as a temporarily difficult time, which may provoke renewed emotions of loss, help the individual to be prepared:

> 'George, the anniversary of Mabel's death is approaching. Have you thought about how you might spend the day? For many people who have faced a major loss like yours, the first anniversary can be a difficult time, often due to the temporary return of overwhelming feelings of loss.'

FINAL PHASE: RECREATING A SENSE OF PURPOSE, LOOKING TO THE FUTURE

This phase is experienced tentatively at first, as individuals fluctuate between the overwhelming emotions of loss and the sense of moving through and on from grief. Usually, individuals become aware of slowly finding enjoyment in past activities, and experiencing increasingly longer periods of time when the death, or other significant loss, is not all-pervasive in their thoughts. The tumult of pain eases, with the raw, stomach-churning feelings of grief episodic, and no longer having the power to dominate life totally. An awareness of feeling relaxed and enjoying life, however short-lived, is experienced once more.

Task of integrating loss

Many writers describing the process of grieving see this phase as one of completion, with the bereaved individual 'letting go' of the significant other who has been lost, allowing life with all its challenges to be pursued again. Worden (1988) writes of the bereaved completing

> any unfinished business with the deceased and being able to say a final goodbye.

For older people, 'letting go' of a significant other, or a long-lived familiar way of life, is extremely difficult. However, during this final phase of grieving, many older people can experience an integration of the loss into their lives, resulting in an acceptance being felt and expressed about what has happened. Achieving some resolution of loss may, nevertheless, provoke a disquieting feeling that crucial parts of a long personal history are slipping out of the individual's grasp. There may be a strong sense that the most purposeful, meaningful and autonomous stages in life have been consigned to the past.

For a number of older people, the resolution of loss is more elusive, making the future difficult to confront. Individuals may appear to be stuck in the second phase of grieving; there may be a constant wish to replay familiar bereavement reminiscences about the significant loss they have experienced. Feelings of despair and loss may remain dominant and intense in expressions of grief. Any suggestion of moving on and looking to the future may be viewed as pointless, and implying disloyalty to the deceased.

Older people with strong social and family supports, and retained autonomy due to good physical and mental health, are likely to be the most successful in integrating loss into their lives. They may also feel more hopeful about developing a new way of being in relation to the world, during this final phase of grieving. In this phase of grief, older people living independently in the community may invest in the future by taking on new responsibilities through voluntary work; developing new interests, or resuming old ones, and/or having more involvement with children and grandchildren.

Supporting older people through this phase of grieving, when there have been multiple losses of spouse, home, familiar way of life, peers and personal physical and mental wellbeing, is very challenging for reminiscence workers. Leick and Davidsen-Nielsen (1991) describe how supporting individuals through the grieving process involves hearing empathetically the expression of isolation and purposelessness, often experienced in this phase, in order that a personal resolution is reached:

> Each person must face a sense of emptiness and meaninglessness in their life and emerge with a personal solution.

Finding a 'personal solution' to grieving that allows them to move on into the future is not always possible for older people. In the face of loss, many feel the best is behind them in life. If a reminiscence worker can empathetically 'be with' older people as such sentiments are expressed, individuals feel accepted and valued. Additionally, if in their present lives older people know they are respected, and that carers have an interest in who they are and what they can offer, it may be possible for them to feel easier about their loss.

Beneficial role of bereavement reminiscence

Bereavement reminiscence can play a role in helping older people express the feelings of loneliness and purposelessness often experienced in this phase of grieving. Reminiscence workers faced with the repetitious recall of bereavement reminiscences may feel that it cannot be helpful to older people. However, there may be a valuable, ongoing contribution that bereavement reminiscence can make to older people's lives. If there is diminishing pain, evident satisfaction, and the maintenance of self-esteem to be observed in the process of repeated recall about someone or *something* that has been lost, then the individual may be utilising bereavement reminiscence in a positive way. It may be a way of regularly engaging the past to revitalise the present and restore emotional strength to cope with an unfamiliar future.

When individuals are faced with the death of a significant other such as a parent, sibling, spouse or peer, the loss experienced is not only of the deceased but often, too, of connections with a particular stage or role in life. As a result, bereavement reminiscence may not be exclusively restricted to recall about the deceased, but may encompass memories associated with other significant people or events in the life history of the bereaved. Therefore, in addition to holding associations and reminders of loss, recall of bereavement reminiscences can provide a repeated rejuvenating effect on individuals through the renewed links with positive, purposeful periods in the past, as illustrated by Madeline's story.

> In quick succession, Madeline experienced the death of two close friends, one of whom she had known since childhood. Both deaths had been sudden, and there had not been the opportunity to see either friend prior to their death. At each loss, Madeline passed quickly through the initial shock phase of grieving, accepting the reality of the death without difficulty. As she entered the second phase of grieving, Madeline initially expressed great sadness and breavement at the loss of her two friends. Bereavement reminiscences centring on specific memories of the friends were recounted repeatedly, often accompanied with tears.
>
> As the weeks passed, bereavement reminiscences focused increasingly only briefly on Madeline's friends; recall widened to include memories not directly related to her friends, but prompted by an often tenuous association with them. Madeline particularly enjoyed recall about her youthful hobby of dancing. The evocative 'memory chain' associated with dancing was stimulated initially by remembering that the mother of one of her deceased friends was a dance instructor.

Madeline's use of bereavement reminiscence illustrates how memories can diverge from an initial painful focus of loss to enjoyable recall about the bereaved individual's past.

THINKING POINT

Can you think of an older person you have talked to following the death of a close friend of theirs? Can you remember their bereavement reminiscences? Did the recall offer comfort through easing the grief of loss and the opportunity to remember positive times from the past?

The way reminiscence workers respond to repeated bereavement reminiscences is crucial in the role they play in offering some alleviation to feelings of loss and purposelessness in the present. As a listener it can be difficult to hear memories time and time again and remain receptive and empathetic. However, knowing that this is one of the strategies older people employ, in an ongoing way, to restore some meaning to the present, may make the effort to remain responsive easier.

Negative bereavement reminiscence

Despite the generally beneficial nature of bereavement reminiscence in older people's lives, a reminiscence worker has to be acutely watchful for signs that this kind of recall is no longer having a positive effect. When, in this final phase of grieving, recall about the deceased is constant, very intense and prompts distress, it may offer some temporary relief to divert the individual's focus of recall, or suggest involvement in a meaningful activity.

Gertrude's experience illustrates how negative responses to grief can complicate the role of positive bereavement reminiscence. Her story illustrates how sensitively diverting individuals from their grief when it is prolonged and/or distressful can be beneficial.

Gertrude was in her eighties when her husband died suddenly after 49 years of marriage. After her husband's death, everywhere in Gertrude's home held poignant memories for her. During the first year after her husband's death, Gertrude regularly shared repeated bereavement reminiscences with her home care. She would also sit for hours opposite a favourite photograph of her husband, talking to it, repeatedly saying how much she missed and still cared for her husband.

The home care became increasingly concerned that, after a year, Gertrude was becoming more, not less distressed, about her loss. 'Talking to' her husband appeared to be making the pain greater for Gertrude, and no longer offered comfort. Eventually, the home care tentatively suggested swapping the photograph of Gertrude's husband for one of her favourite grandson. Gertrude appeared relieved by the suggestion; her grief slowly became less all-consuming and the photograph of her grandson gave her permission to focus again on the present, providing a balance to her loss. Gertrude later told a friend, 'It was so simple, but without the home care's suggestion about the photograph, I would never have started to accept my husband's death.'

Search for meaning

Reminiscence workers when working with older people in the later phases of grieving will be faced with their struggle to find meaning in the future. This search for meaning is painful for individuals to express, and difficult for reminiscence workers to hear. 'Being with' an older person; and offering empathetic acceptance as they put words to this void, is very supportive. Once individuals have explored their feelings about lack of purpose or meaning in their lives, it can be helpful to tentatively look with them at whether there is anything or anyone that eases these feelings and makes life seem a little better, even for a short time. Additionally, previous reminiscence work with the individual may have indicated interests and activities enjoyed in the past that could offer some pleasure if resumed in the present. Enid's story shows how an older person can be helped to find enjoyment after bereavement.

In her late eighties, Enid had experienced moving to a nursing home as the last of many losses in her recent past. She spoke often of having so little that gave her pleasure. Many of Enid's bereavement reminiscences about her home centred around feelings of missing being able to sit looking at her garden.

Enid's room in the home overlooked the car-park, and to restore the opportunity for Enid to enjoy a garden again, it was suggested that she could be helped to the conservatory to sit and look at the garden whenever she wanted. Enid's smile communicated her evident pleasure at this suggestion, and she took to sitting for long periods in the conservatory. As staff came to appreciate how much Enid enjoyed the garden, she was asked to choose a favourite plant to be grown near the conservatory for her to enjoy.

The value of reviving a past interest to create pleasure-in-the-moment for individuals is illustrated in the enjoyment Enid gained from renewing her love of gardens. Returning small pleasures in this way cannot offer a panacea to the pain of loss and accompanying sense of purposelessness. But showing an interest in an individual's uniqueness sends a powerful, comforting message of their continuing value to others. In this way, a small counter to the emptiness of the present is provided.

Responding to bereavement reactions in the final phase

- Empathising with the magnitude of change and loss experienced by older people moving to residential care validates their feelings. It may be difficult for older people to share these feelings with relatives who may feel a mixture of guilt and relief following the admission:

  'Enid, I know it is very difficult for you to share your feelings of loss with your daughter, as she feels responsible for persuading you to move to the home. Giving up your home is a major loss and change. Learning to live with others, experiencing reduced independence and a complete change in your way of life, is very hard and takes time to adjust to.'

- Communicating continuing interest to an older person about rehearing favourite memories connected with the deceased promotes the restorative value of bereavement reminiscence in an individual's life:

  'Yes Madeline, you have told me before about the first time you met your friend but that doesn't matter, your enjoyment in remembering is good to see.'

- Accepting non-judgementally feelings of emptiness and purposelessness expressed by older people in this phase of grieving acknowledges and respects individuals' feelings. Having a responsive person hear these feelings may offer some relief in itself: the individual is shown that they are not totally alone. By acknowledging and expressing emptiness and purposelessness, the individual may be able, at a later stage, to move on through their grief and regain some pleasure in life:

  'Beatrice, your question about what purpose is there left for you now that your husband has died, makes the world sound an empty place for you at the moment. It may help to tell me some more about how you feel.'

COMPLICATED GRIEF REACTIONS

The grieving process, following bereavement, is a major emotional and physical assault on older people's equilibrium, and is too overwhelming for some individuals to cope with. A minority of older people may respond to their loss by exhibiting complicated grief reactions, which cause concern for their carers. It is advisable in these situations to obtain a specialist's view.

Complicated grief reactions can be difficult to identify, as the normal grieving process is an individual one that shows a range of reactions and a wide time differences in 'recovery' from loss. Reactions that may indicate a complicated reaction to grief include:

- **Intensification of grief:** This is when the expression of distress about a loss, rather than easing becomes more intense, frequent and all consuming as the months pass. Heightened grief may also be accompanied by strong feelings of guilt, suicidal feelings and/or self-neglect.

- **Long-term denial of loss:** Persistent and long-term denial of loss results in an unshakeable belief that the deceased is still alive: the deceased may be constantly referred to as if they are in the house or out of the home, carrying on with normal everyday tasks. Food for the deceased may be bought and prepared, as previously. Conversations may be recalled as if they have taken place with the deceased. In addition, individuals may show a general disconnection from everyday reality. Such a complicated grief reaction may indicate a mental health difficulty; individuals experiencing dementia prior to a major loss may be unable at any point to comprehend and absorb its reality.

- **Postponed grief:** This occurs when an individual exhibits a minimal or complete absence of response to loss, acting as if nothing untoward has happened, living life as normal. This response is not related to the detached feelings of normal early grief, but is a deliberate attempt to continue to avoid or delay the pain of loss. Practical pressures resulting from the loss may leave the individual with little energy or time to face the onslaught of grief. Alternatively, individuals may feel that they must be strong for the sake of others, and put their own pain on hold until the future. Such postponement of grief usually leads to an accumulation of emotion that finds release at a later time, possibly overwhelming the individual with its intensity.

  Listening and responding appropriately to older people experiencing bereavement is very demanding; lack of time and/or confidence in skills can make it difficult for carers to cope. Support in these instances may be available from the voluntary or statutory sectors: CRUSE is a national organisation in Britain working with bereaved people. There are local branches throughout the country offering training for volunteers and professionals. Volunteers trained by CRUSE offer one-to-one and groupwork counselling support to the bereaved. In some situations, social workers and community nurses may also be able to offer short-term bereavement support.

Summary Points

Promoting One-to-One Reminiscence

- One-to-one reminiscence work holds the possibility of focusing on many areas of an individual's past: social and personal aspects of everyday life; bereavement events related to the loss of someone or *something* significant; preferences and interests that afforded pleasure and comfort.
- Life-history work for individuals promotes continuity between the past, present and future; celebrates life events; helps acknowledge and, in some instances, come to terms with unresolved issues from the past.
- The variation in format and content of life-story books reflects the uniqueness of the experience of each older person.
- The impact of loss on older people's lives is felt not only following the death of a significant other, but also when coming to terms with the loss of *something* precious.
- Cultural and religious beliefs and traditions offer support to many older people facing bereavement. Whatever beliefs individuals hold, the emotions and tasks of grieving will be similar.
- One-to-one reminiscence work with people with dementia affords opportunities to maintain and renew relevant and personalised links with the past, while maintaining and extending social relationships in the present.
- Sensitive responses to bereavement reminiscences within life-story work counter society's undermining devaluation of older people's grief.

Training Activities

Activity 1 / 1

1

Countering Stereotypes: Promoting Personhood

MAIN TEXT REFERENCES: INTRODUCTION, CHAPTER 1

Purpose

1 To become more aware of personal and societal attitudes towards ageing and older people generally.

2 To consider how negative stereotyping reduces the ability to view older people as individuals with different needs and unique histories.

3 To consider how reminiscence work can help carers promote a personhood approach to care practices, by increasing awareness of the individuality of older people.

What to do

- Prior to training session, if possible, to facilitate discussion, locate writings, poems or newspaper photographs that illustrate negative and positive stereotypes of older people. Alternatively, the two poems on page 136 could be used to stimulate discussion about getting older.

- Trainer starts the session by sharing with the group the purpose of the activity as outlined above.

- Continue by discussing how negative stereotypes of older people influence patterns of caring. Look at how stereotypes can create preconceived expectations of behaviour and needs, making it more difficult to recognise, acknowledge and respond to the uniqueness or personhood of each older person.

- Read out the two poems on page 136 on getting older or your own examples, to stimulate some thoughts and discussion about ageing. How do the ideas expressed match or disagree with the group's view of getting older?

Activity 1 / 2

1

Nobody Grows Old

Nobody grows old by merely living a number of years
People grow old by deserting their ideals
You are as young as your self-confidence,
As old as your fear,
As young as your hope,
As old as your despair.
In the central place of every heart, there is a recording chamber.
So long as it receives messages of beauty, hope, cheer and courage,
So long are you young.
When the wires are all down, and your heart is covered with the
Snows of pessimism and the ice of cynicism,
Then and only then, are you grown OLD.

DOUGLAS MACARTHUR

Getting Older

The first surprise: I like it.
Whatever happens now, some things
That used to terrify have not:

I didn't die young, for instance. Or lose my only love.
My three children never had to run away from anyone.
Don't tell me this gratitude is complacent
We all approach the edge of the same blackness
Which for me is silent.

Knowing as much sharpens my delight in January freesia,
Hot coffee, winter sunlight.
So we say as we lie close on some gentle occasion; every
Day won from such darkness is a celebration.

ELAINE FEINSTEIN

Activity 1 / 3

1

- Ask the group to brainstorm a list of all the words, terms or sayings that relate to ageing or older people. Some examples are shown in the following diagram, to use as prompts with the group.

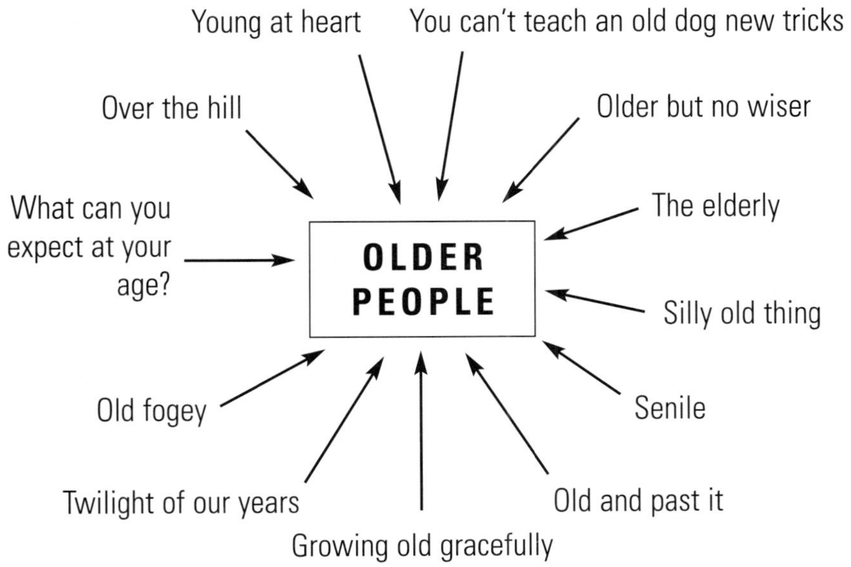

- When the group has exhausted suggestions, look together at how many of the comments about getting older are negative rather than positive.

- Take a few of the suggestions and encourage the group to look at the general expectations of older people that these create, in terms of behaviour, interests, motivation, needs and hopes.

To sum up

Point out how negative and limiting expectations of ageing can affect personal attitudes towards older people. Restrictive stereotypes may influence carers to lower their ambitions for older people. Individuality illustrated by different needs, interests and backgrounds may not be fully recognised and respected. Point out that reminiscence work offers a counter to the restricting views encouraged by stereotypes of older people. It strongly illustrates the diverse and unique backgrounds of the individuals whom carers live or work with, encouraging carers to concentrate more on individuals' histories, personalities and needs. In short, reminiscence work promotes a personhood approach to care practices.

Activity 2 / 1

2

Valuing Older People through Reminiscence Work

MAIN TEXT REFERENCES: CHAPTERS 1 & 2

Purpose

1 To become more aware of what older people view as valuable in their lives.

2 To increase empathy for older people's needs.

3 To look at how reminiscence work can offer value to older people, by creating increased feelings of self-worth and purpose.

What to do

- Trainer starts the session by sharing the purpose of the activity as outlined above.

- Continue by asking the group to brainstorm the areas of their lives that they value and enjoy. Ask for general words, such as 'home', 'family', 'friends', 'holidays', 'going out', 'possessions'.

Variation: Prior to the training session, ask group members to select an object or photograph to bring along that represents something they value and enjoy in their lives. For example, a photograph of their house, garden or favourite holiday destination.

- Ask the group to break into pairs and discuss, in turn, the following value statements. Which ones do they feel apply to them? Ask individuals to say a little about each value statement they feel is relevant to them. Can they think of any other more personally appropriate value statements?

  – I value my close family, whom I live with or see regularly.

  – It is important to me that I have friends I talk to and see regularly.

Activity 2 / 2

2

- I value time in my home to do what I want, when and how I please.
- I enjoy doing things spontaneously, without planning or always following a routine.

◆ In the large group, encourage a general discussion about the value statements. Did the group largely think the statements were appropriate to their lives? Did anyone have any difficulty with any of the statements? Could anyone think of more appropriate personal value statements?

◆ Look together at how individuals generally gain a sense of being valuable in the world, through belonging to social systems, such as family, friends and work.

◆ Ask the large group to brainstorm how they feel generally when they experience a sense of being valued in their lives.

◆ Ask the group to keep these thoughts in mind about the areas that they value in their lives and how it feels to be valued. To move the focus to older people, ask group members to think about a person they care for, and to recall the individual's room, their possessions, activities, hobbies, and relatives and friends who may visit.

◆ Ask each individual to write four value statements on behalf of the older person they have been thinking about. Suggest working with previous partners to discuss the statements.

◆ Back in the large group, discuss generally how easy or difficult it was to write these statements. Was it hard to think of four appropriate ones? Would one or two people volunteer to have their statements written up for the group to discuss? How do these statements contrast with the personal statements of group members at the start of the activity? Are they more restricted? Do they cover different areas or similar ones? Do group members think the older person would be happy with these value statements? Are there areas in their lives that older people they care for would like more choice about?

Activity 2 / 3

2

To sum up

Encourage the group to think about how a broad, regular reminiscence programme can be very valuable in making older people's lives more sociable, by increasing the quality of communication with carers; offering a change in routine; an emphasis for a time on social as opposed to physical care. In addition, reminiscence activities provide the opportunity to rekindle older people's past interests.

Activity 3 / 1

3

Making Listening Matter

MAIN TEXT REFERENCE: CHAPTER 2

Purpose

1 To emphasize the importance of communication as one of the key skills in reminiscence work.

2 To recognise situations where effective listening is important.

3 To practise different styles of listening to reinforce the value of developing appropriate verbal and non-verbal listening skills.

4 To improve communication by understanding the difference between effective and ineffective listening skills.

What to do

- Trainer begins the session by outlining the purpose of the session as outlined above.

- Continue by asking the group to brainstorm situations where it is important to use effective listening skills. Draw up three columns covering different categories of listening situations as shown. Encourage the group to think about personal, social and work relationships where there is a need to both listen well to others and be listened to. Examples of situations in each category are given in the table below.

Activity 3 / 2

3

Personal situations when we need to listen	***Work situations when we need to listen***	***Professionals who we want to listen to us***
Talking to children about difficulties at school.	An older person expressing regrets about having to give up their home or the death of a close relative or friend.	Doctors
Talking to a partner having problems finding a job.	A colleague who has a grievance about work.	Solicitors
Talking to a bereaved friend.		Teachers
		Supervisors

- Point out to the group that although the use of effective listening skills will improve general everyday communication, there are certain personal and work situations where their use is essential to ensure that thoughts and feelings can be expressed and responded to well.

- Develop several of the examples given by the group of where effective listening is important. Promote discussion of any difficulties that group members experience in hearing and responding in different listening situations. Look at examples where individuals have felt they have not been listened to well, and examples of where listening has been sensitive. Highlight the contrasting attitudes and ways of listening, in order to emphasize effective listening skills.

- Ask the group to brainstorm how it feels to be listened to well. Suggestions may include: 'accepted; 'eased tension'; 'helped to make a decision'; 'understood'; 'respected and valued'.

- Continue by completing the following pair exercises, in different listening styles, to enable the group to determine the most effective style.

Activity 3 / 3

3

Note: The first three listening styles employ techniques that are strongly inappropriate in creating an effective listening atmosphere, and may evoke humour in both the listener and speaker as they follow the exercises through. In contrast, the fourth listening style reflects appropriate and effective use of listening skills.

- Ask the group to split into pairs, and to alternate as listener and speaker in each exercise. For the purpose of the exercises, individuals are asked to talk, for a short time, about an everyday incident that has annoyed them recently.

  Exercise A: Speaker is seated and listener stands behind the chair. Speaker talks for up to two minutes about an annoying situation with the listener saying nothing. The pair reverse roles and repeat the exercise.

  Exercise B: Speaker is seated with listener standing in front of them. For up to two minutes the speaker develops further the annoying incident they have experienced. This time the listener says nothing, but shuffles about and looks away from the speaker. The pair reverse roles and repeat the exercise.

  Exercise C: Speaker is seated and listener sits to the side, with arms folded and legs crossed, staring ahead. The speaker continues to talk about their chosen incident for a further minute, with the listener interrupting regularly saying they need to leave in a second to finish a task. The pair reverse roles and repeat the exercise.

  Exercise D: For the final part of the exercise listener and speaker are seated opposite each other; at the same level; close but not invading each other's territory. Listener adopts an open posture; maintains eye contact without staring; avoids fidgeting; nods to show understanding; avoids interrupting, except to acknowledge the difficulty of the situation. The speaker takes up to five minutes to conclude their recall of an annoying incident, looking at any ways they feel the situation could have been handled differently. The pair reverse roles and repeat the exercise.

- Continue the exercise by asking the group to comment on the four different listening styles. Which one did they find most effective as a listener, and as a speaker?

Activity 3 / 4 3

- From the observations made in the exercise, ask the group to brainstorm in two columns effective non-verbal and verbal listening skills. Skills highlighted by the group could include those shown in the following table.

Effective non-verbal listening skills	***Effective verbal listening skills***
Good attention	Being clear about available time
Sitting opposite at same level	Acknowledging depth of difficulty by expressing empathy for individual
Sitting near without being invasive	Open questions, encouraging further exploration of difficulty
Open, relaxed posture	Encouraging and allowing expression of feelings and thoughts
Maintaining eye contact without staring	Not interrupting
Nodding	
Giving time	
Showing interest	
Not fidgeting	

To sum up

Emphasize the key role that communication, based on effective listening, plays in promoting sensitive reminiscence work. Knowledge of, and confidence in, the use of effective listening skills, enhances a carer's ability to hear and respond to the emotive thoughts and feelings expressed by older people during the reminiscence process.

Activity 4 / 1

4

How it Feels to Reminisce

MAIN TEXT REFERENCES: CHAPTERS 2, 4 & 7

Purpose

1 To illustrate the process of reminiscence, particularly how memories are evoked.

2 To experience how it feels to remember and share memories one-to-one and in a group.

3 To increase feelings of self-worth by naming and valuing carer's own past.

4 To experience the enjoyment of reminiscing, to encourage use of this work with older people.

What to do

- Share the purpose of the activity as outlined above.
- Read out the following quotes to act as triggers to stimulate group members' recall of schooldays:

  'My best friend at school was Betty. Our favourite game at playtime was "kiss chase" with the boys, but we had to be careful the teachers didn't catch us.'

  'My worst teacher at school was Mrs Tate; she was so strict and would often cane the boys. I remember my first day in her class, and crying because I couldn't copy my name properly on to my blue name card.'

- Ask the group to begin to think of their earliest memory of school.
- Encourage each group member to take a few minutes to think back to school days. Suggest that memories could be recalled about a certain teacher, classroom or friend, or any other area of school life.

Activity 4 / 2

4

- After five minutes, or longer if required, ask the group to pair up and take it in turns to listen to each other's memories (remind about effective listening skills in Activity 3). Reassure group members who found their school days difficult to recall that not all themes are equally evocative for everyone. Point out that older people too find some themes more personally specific and interesting than others.
- Emphasize that there may be some memories that individuals find difficult to share: school days for most people have happy and sad associations. Point out that all themes in reminiscence work have the potential for prompting happy and sad recall. Reminiscence workers need to be sensitive to older people who experience painful feelings associated with past memories.
- After 10–15 minutes, bring everyone back to the large group. Encourage a sharing of group members' memories.
- Ask if anyone recalled the feelings associated with going to school for the first time as a small child.
- Make links between common memories around school, and encourage positive feelings about being able to remember the past and sharing this with others.
- Ask how it felt to reminiscence and share memories with others. What was observed about the process of reminiscing? Encourage comments about whether it was easy or not to remember schooldays; how effective the 'trigger' was in stimulating memory; if one memory lead easily to another; whether memories went off at a tangent; if there was general enjoyment in sharing memories with an interested listener.

To sum up

Emphasize that, when reminiscing, older people experience the same process of recall as group members, with memories being evoked through the use of triggers related to the chosen theme. The most effective triggers are those that are personally relevant to the individual. In group reminiscence sessions, individuals are also triggered to remember by the stimulus of memories of peers.

Activity 5 / 1

5

The Role of Background Information in Reminiscence Work

MAIN TEXT REFERENCES: CHAPTERS 2 & 3

MATERIALS NEEDED: Copies of the Group Member's Profile Form.

Purpose

1 To emphasize the value of gaining background information on potential group members prior to the start of group reminiscence sessions, to ensure that: individuals are referred to in a way they are comfortable with; appropriate themes with personal interest are used; individuals feel their past is valued by the reminiscence worker promoting confidence in the reminiscence process generally.

2 To promote familiarity with the use of the Group Member's Profile Form as a tool for gaining and recording background information about group members.

3 To increase awareness of the potentially sensitive nature of information gained through the reminiscence process.

What to do

- Share the purpose of the activity as outlined above.
- Ask the group to split into pairs, and remind them about the listening skills covered in Activity 3. Ask individuals to take clear turns in sharing information about their names with their partner: Do they know how they came to be called by their name? Do they like their name? Is there a name they have always wanted to be called or feel is more appropriate to their personality? Were they, or are they still called by a nickname? Do they like or dislike the nickname?
- Promote large group discussion around the pairs' exercise on names. Encourage group members to share the story of their name, pointing out an individual's name is an important part of their identity. Emphasize that it is important to be

Activity 5 / 2

5

certain that an older person is being called by the name they are familiar with, which may not be the name shown on official forms. Remind the group that name origin, as with other personal information, needs to be gained with sensitivity to potential painful areas of older people's lives, which may include death in childbirth of mother; being raised by grandparents or other relatives; lack of knowledge of birth parents; adoption or fostering or life in the workhouse as a child.

- Encourage group members to share any instances when they have been referred to by a disliked nickname or incorrect name: how did this make them feel? Have they any examples of using the wrong name with older people they care for? If so, what was the effect?

- Look with group members at how additional background information about individuals can be collected by completing the Group Member's Profile Form, which emphasizes the importance of finding out background knowledge about older people's past and present enjoyment of special places, events and achievements.

- To illustrate the value of the Group Member's Profile Form in obtaining valuable background information, ask group members to complete the following sections on the form, with a partner:

  – Name the places and events of special importance in your life

  – The reasons for their importance

  – What I am proud to have achieved

- Encourage individuals, when completing the above questions, to think about what significant events they would feel it important for a group leader to know if they were attending a reminiscence group.

- Encourage large group discussion of the information shared in the pairs exercise. Did individuals find it easy and valuable to think about the special times and achievements in their lives? Encourage positive feelings about events and achievements shared; point out that this acknowledging and celebration of individuals' lives is one of the key tasks of reminiscence workers.

Activity 5 / 3

5

To sum up

Look at how the exercises in this activity have helped to illustrate, through personal involvement, some key points about the value of information-gathering in the reminiscence process. Highlight how requesting information about the history of an individual's name can provide a good opening question when collecting background details about an older person. Additionally, being clear about how an individual wishes to be referred to shows valuing of the older person and helps maintain their sense of identity. Gathering information on older people's special times further helps promotion of a personhood approach to care through the valuing and celebration of the uniqueness of individuals.

Activity 6 / 1

6

Illustrating the Value of Themes and Triggers in Reminiscence Work

MAIN TEXT REFERENCE: CHAPTER 6

MATERIALS NEEDED: Selection of triggers relating to a broad range of themes.

Purpose

1 To highlight and emphasize the role that themes and triggers play in reminiscence groupwork.

2 To emphasize the very wide range of themes and triggers available for use in reminiscence work.

3 To highlight how personal involvement and interest in particular themes and triggers can stimulate the process of remembering for older people.

4 To illustrate how knowledge about the background of older people attending reminiscence groups is valuable in helping to identify appropriate themes and related triggers.

What to do

- Share with the group the purpose of the activity as outlined above.
- Ask the group to brainstorm all the general themes they can think of that could be used in reminiscence work. Encourage the group to decide if any of these themes provide older people with an opportunity for taking part in a hands-on activity.
- One example of a hands-on activity related to the theme of eating and drinking could be based around the preparation of an old-fashioned afternoon tea party, involving the group in making a traditional cake and a cup of tea using old china cups, tea leaves and a crock teapot. Point out that taking part in a hands-on activity, which has a reminiscence base, is often particularly effective in stirring memories.

Activity 6 / 2

6

- Select two or three themes from those suggested by the group and ask them to think of a selection of triggers that relate to the chosen themes.
- Alternatively, if the trainer has a set of triggers available as a resource for this activity, use these to encourage the group to think which themes the triggers relate to. Remind the group of the wide range of triggers that can be used in the work, and the importance of ensuring varying sensory appeal. Additionally, triggers should appeal to all cultures represented in the group.
- Ask group members to think which one of the themes listed holds particular interest for them. Split the group into pairs and remind individuals about taking clear turns. Ask group members to share with their partner, for about five minutes each, the theme they have chosen, and a memory related to the theme, either from childhood or young adulthood. Emphasize to group members the potential sensitivity of some themes, and ask individuals for the purpose of this exercise to focus on a positive memory.
- Bring group members back to the large group and ask individuals to share which theme listed provoked memories for them. Stress that they do not have to recall the memory they shared with the large group unless they want to. Point out that generally older people too, find it easier to share more personal memories on a one-to-one basis than in a group.
- Ask group members to think about an older person they care for or have cared for; from the background knowledge available about this individual ask them to select a theme and related triggers that would be of interest to them. Discuss the chosen themes and triggers in the large group, particularly concentrating on why it was felt individuals would enjoy the identified themes and triggers.

To sum up

Highlight the variety of themes and triggers the group were able to identify as appropriate for use in reminiscence work. Point out that reminiscence work is illuminated for older people by feeling a personal connection with themes and triggers. The effectiveness of triggers is further enhanced if they offer appeal to a variety of senses, and the different cultural backgrounds of group members.

Activity 7 / 1

7

Promoting Reminiscence Work with Minority Cultures

MAIN TEXT REFERENCE: CHAPTER 6

MATERIALS NEEDED: Quotes from older people on the subject of emigration, see also variation below.

Purpose

1 To highlight the expectations and hopes of people from minority cultures when adopting a new homeland.

2 To become more aware of the impact of immigration and cultural influences on people from minority cultures.

3 To increase knowledge of appropriate culturally specific themes and triggers that enhance the reminiscence experience for people from minority cultures.

What to do

- Share the purpose of the activity as outlined above.

- As a large group, brainstorm remembered thoughts, fears and hopes experienced when making a major personal life change, such as moving schools, jobs or homes. Suggest that individuals recall their first days in a new school or job, moving house to a different town or into the country, or emigrating to a foreign country. Ask group members to choose a change that had a strong impact on their lives and involved meeting new people and/or moving somewhere different.

- List the fears and hopes shared by the group in separate columns and promote a discussion about similarities and differences in experience, bringing out detail about how individuals coped with their fears, and how far their hopes were fulfilled.

Activity 7 / 2

7

- Ask group members from their experience of talking to people from minority cultures either in work or personal situations (relatives or friends), to recall their comments about the experience of immigration. List any fears or hopes shared about this life changing event and contrast with the group members' comments earlier in the activity.

Variation: Reading out quotes from personal experiences can also stimulate discussion of the challenges met by older people when they initially immigrated to a new homeland. One source is the Age Exchange publication, *A Place to Stay – Memories of Pensioners from Many Lands.*

- Bring out in large group discussion the likely feelings arising from the thwarted hopes in achieving good jobs and homes, experienced by many people from minority cultures on arrival in Britain. Point out the difficulty immigrants would have faced in coping with personal and institutional racism, and language barriers. Explain that the feelings experienced would have been made all the more difficult and complex by the hopeful expectations held by immigrants arriving in Britain; hopeful expectations that arose from the positive British government immigration policy in operation in the years immediately following the Second World War.

- Emphasize that adopting a new homeland, with all its challenges in work, housing, and building new social links, is one of the most major life-changing events that can be experienced by an individual. Point out that by raising personal awareness about fears and hopes that accompany changes in living or working situations, it is possible to develop greater empathy for individuals who experienced immigration with its major changes and challenges.

- Ask the large group to think about planning reminiscence groupwork with people from a minority culture within their unit: how could the group reaffirm cultural traditions and celebrations of older people from the minority culture?

- Brainstorm all the religious or other cultural events past and present celebrated by older people from the minority culture within the unit. Discuss whether these events are currently marked in the unit. How could a reminiscence group acknowledge and celebrate these special cultural events?

Activity 7 / 3

7

- Encourage the group to think about appropriate, culturally specific triggers relating to one of these celebrations. Appropriate suggestions would include reading out published quotes from older people about their memories of past celebrations; photographs of events, past and present; preparing and eating traditional food; looking at or wearing traditional dress; obtaining or making appropriate decorations; attending local community celebrations, or bringing local groups into the unit to share in the celebrations.

To sum up

Emphasize that immigration to a new homeland is one of the most challenging life events individuals can face; developing empathy for older people grown old in an adopted land helps to promote a positive, valuing reminiscence experience. Using reminiscence work to reaffirm the value of cultural traditions and celebrations shows respect for, and interest in, older people from minority cultures. Promoting the recording of memories in older people's first language helps to preserve and transmit cultural history for their children, grandchildren, and the wider community.

Activity 8 / 1

8

Promoting Reminiscence Work with People with Dementia

MAIN TEXT REFERENCE: CHAPTER 5

MATERIALS NEEDED: General selection of sensory triggers. For example, hand massage oil, compilation tape of songs from the past, mothballs, leaf tea, flowers, and traditional cakes or biscuits.

Purpose

1 To develop greater understanding about how people with dementia feel about their world, and the role reminiscence work can play in the maintenance of the personhood of individuals.

2 To extend knowledge of the kinds of triggers that hold particular appeal for people with dementia.

3 To reflect on the role that group reminiscence work or a reminiscence-based activity programme can play in the lives of people with dementia.

What to do

- Share with the group the purpose of the activity, as outlined above.
- Ask the group to start by throwing a soft ball to each other. When the ball is caught, the group member who threw it has to say the individual's name, and a quality that is liked about the person as a colleague.
- Encourage group members to share how it felt to hear positive comments about themselves. Emphasize to the group that this way of opening sessions, with leaders making a valuing comment to each individual as the ball is thrown to members of the group, is a warm way to begin group reminiscence sessions with people with dementia. It promotes personhood by showing individuals that they are valued for their distinct personalities and interests.

Activity 8 / 2

8

- With the group, look at how it would be possible to gain some insight into how people with dementia view their world through personal experiences: small incidents happen in everyone's daily life that provide fleeting glimpses of the frustrations and difficulties felt by people with dementia.

- Quote some common examples of behaviour that provoke temporary reactions of frustration, confusion and embarrassment in people who do not have dementia:
  - Going into a room and forgetting why you are there
  - After moving furniture around at home, continuing, perhaps for some time, to go back to where items of furniture were originally

- Encourage the group to give examples of their own similar behaviour, and write these up. Some more examples are:
  - Forgetting the name of someone, or a object
  - Having to ask someone to remind you where 'the safe place', in which you put an object, is

This part of the activity often provokes a lot of laughter, and sometimes relief, as individuals realise that other people also experience everyday forgetfulness. Ask group members to recall how they feel on these occasions. It is likely that group members describing their feelings and responses in these situations will refer to irritation, embarrassment, laughter, exasperation and annoyance. Point out to the group that how they feel when experiencing these inconsequential incidents provides a small insight into how people with dementia feel about their world.

Explain that such incidents, for individuals not experiencing dementia, are irritating happenings often arising out of having too many things to think about at once. These incidents do not have the ability to prevent individuals relating to others or taking part in the world generally. The major difference in the experience of people with dementia is that the emphasis in their lives is constantly on forgetting; not recognising once-familiar people or places; not recalling where they live; increasingly finding it harder to do simple tasks. For people with dementia, relating to a world that is constantly changing and making often mystifying demands, becomes maze-like in its complexity.

Activity 8 / 3

8

- Ask group members to think about a person with dementia they care for, and what reactions and feelings they show that illustrate how they are trying to cope with their changing lives. Write up some of these reactions and feelings, making comparisons with those felt by group members when faced with their own puzzling behaviour.

The reactions and feelings experienced by people with dementia are likely to be similar, but far more regular, long-lasting, intense, distressing and harder to dispel. Additionally, these feelings experienced may result in individuals experiencing dementia to actively 'look' for a secure figure from the past to offer comfort in their distress.

- Encourage group members to begin to think how reminiscence work with people with dementia can offer insight and information, enabling communication paths to grow between carers and people with dementia. In this way, a counter is provided to the progressively disorientating effects of dementia.

- Ask group members to split into pairs, and to share ideas about how reminiscence work in small groups, or a reminiscence-based activity programme, could help an individual they are caring for. It may be easiest to think of ideas under three headings:

  1. *Pleasure-in-the-moment:* What accompanied activity, object, or music, gives or could be promoted to give pleasure-in-the-moment to the individual?

  2. *Sensory triggers:* From background information about the individual, is there a personal sensory trigger that would help prompt recall?

  3. *Reminiscence-based activity:* What does the individual like to do to relax that could be incorporated into a reminiscence-based activity programme to create a quiet time?

- Bring the group back together, and ask them to share the ideas for promoting reminiscence work with people with dementia whom they care for. Write up the ideas to promote group discussion. If examples of triggers are available, use these to widen discussion about appropriate sensory triggers.

Activity 8 / 4

8

To sum up

Look at how the activity has concentrated on building up a greater insight into how people with dementia view their world. By each group member focusing on one individual, it will have been possible to identify how reminiscence work can build communication paths between carers and individuals with dementia, through the use of personal triggers and meaningful sources of pleasure-in-the-moment.

Activity 9 / 1

9

Developing Life History Work

MAIN TEXT REFERENCES: CHAPTERS 5 & 7

Purpose

1 To develop awareness of the value of life-history work.

2 To look at the various ways life-history work can be recorded.

3 To consider how the use of personally specific triggers promotes the process of recall in life-history work.

4 To promote awareness of the ongoing value of life-story records.

What to do

- Share with the group the purpose of the activity, as outlined above.
- Ask the group to brainstorm what they feel the value of one-to-one life-history work is for older people and their carers. To help stimulate ideas, ask group members to think about what they gain from sharing thoughts about their own past with a friend. Alternatively, ask them to focus on an older person they have spent time with talking about the past and to think what that individual gained from the experience.
- Write up the group ideas in two columns, the first showing the value to older people, and the second the gains to carers. Ideas to prompt are shown in the table on the next page.

Activity 9 / 2

9

Value to older people	Value to carers
Enjoyment	Pleasure
Enhanced self-awareness and self-esteem	Enhanced background knowledge
Improved relationship with carer	Increase of empathy
Appreciation and celebration of life events	Improved relationship
'Laying ghosts' from the past	Job satisfaction
Support in grieving process	Ideas for pleasure-in-the-moment work
Support for terminally ill individuals	Chance to involve relatives
Strength to cope with here-and-now	Chance to help people with dementia retain their sense of identity
Chance to sum up attitudes to past and present	Supports and develops personhood approach to care practices
Preserve memories in form of a life-story record	

- Encourage discussion of the values listed, highlighting where gains have value for older people and carers alike.

- Ask the group to split into small groups and discuss any life-history work they have undertaken, and if life-story records were made. Ask each group to list the various kinds of life-story records produced. Remind group members that not all older people want a record of their life history, and that this does not diminish its value.

- Bring the groups back together and list all the different forms of life-story records made. Examples could include: life-story books; annotated photo albums or boards; audio or video recordings; family trees; memory boxes.

- Promote discussion about the experience of the group in using different styles of life-history recording. Point out that the variation in format and content of

Activity 9 / 3

9

life-story records reflects the unique experience of each older person undertaking the work. Acknowledging and celebrating differences within life-story work helps promote personhood of care for each individual.

- Ask the group to share how life-story books were compiled. For example, were photographs, maps, drawings, favourite pictures, poems or other items included?
- Point out that when compiling life-story records, focusing only on one life stage, possibly childhood, with people experiencing dementia can be very effective: 'windows' of memory often remain intact about the long-term past, and tapping into this recall provides a lot of pleasure for people with dementia.
- In addition, if subsequently these memories are lost, the life-story record provides an effective way of keeping the individual in touch with this period in their life.
- Promote discussion in the large group about the use of triggers in evoking memories in life-history work. Point out that background knowledge can suggest effective triggers. For example, if it is known that an individual's husband or father was a baker, photographs or artefacts connected with the trade could be obtained to stimulate memories. Do group members have any examples of triggers used in their life-story work with individuals?
- Discuss in the large group the ongoing value of life-story records in providing a focus for one-to-one work with individuals; new information about events happening in the present can be added where appropriate. What, if any, is the group members' experience of the ongoing use of life-story records with individuals?

To sum up

Emphasize that life-history work, recorded or not, has value for older people and carers alike. There are many ways of recording details of an individual's life. Personally specific triggers are very effective in stimulating and enlivening the process of recall. Life-story records offer a focus for extending the continuity of individuals' past and present lives.

Activity 10 / 1

10

The Role of Loss in Reminiscence Work

MAIN TEXT REFERENCE: CHAPTER 7

Purpose

1 To increase awareness about the kinds of losses faced by older people.

2 To enhance understanding of what helps and hinders in communicating with older people facing loss in their lives.

3 To consider the role of bereavement reminiscences in one-to-one work.

What to do

- Share the purpose of the activity with the group, as outlined above.
- Look with the large group at how the impact of loss on older people's lives is felt from both death of significant people and the loss of *something* precious, for example, a familiar way of life. Point out that how past losses have been coped with, present support systems, and the effect of multiple sequential loss on older people, are all factors that influence how present loss is experienced by individuals.
- Promote a group brainstorm of significant losses in older people's lives that are distinct from death. The kinds of losses to highlight include:
  - Independence through mental and physical health difficulties
  - Home and possessions through admission to care
  - Choice and freedom when living in care regimes
  - Reduced contact with neighbours, friends and family
  - Inability to continue caring for a garden or pet

Activity 10 / 2

10

- Look together at this list of losses, and consider their impact on individuals. Point out that reminiscence work often highlights older people's feelings about the loss of *something* precious in their lives. Bereavement reminiscences about the loss of past homes, physical independence or a former familiar way of life, are often expressed during one-to-one work. Reminiscence workers need to acknowledge the significance of this kind of loss to individuals, and view connected bereavement reminiscences as part of the process of coming to terms with the loss.

- Encourage a group discussion about what hinders and helps when working with individuals sharing bereavement reminiscences connected to loss associated with death or other significant loss.

- The use of platitudes is one hindrance that it is valuable to highlight. Explain that platitudes are well-known set responses made to people who have been bereaved, and that they may have the effect of blocking expression of feelings; devaluing the extent of grief experienced; offering a response inappropriate in terms of the phase of grieving currently experienced by the individual; protecting the carer from personal fears related to death, or general fears about their own or a relative's future.

- Ask the group to brainstorm some familiar platitudes. Encourage individuals to think about the message implied in these and similar responses, and how they may block expressions of grief.

- Take two or three of the platitudes, and look closely at their meaning and appropriateness. For example, 'time heals everything': time is one factor in the recovery from grief, but the use of this platitude – particularly during the early days and weeks of an individual's grief – could be seen as a way of denying, and devaluing the pain of loss. Additionally, in the early phase of bereavement, the idea of being able to get over a major loss, may be viewed by the individual as inconceivable and disloyal.

- Another example of a platitude is 'Don't be sad, death come to us all.' By stating the obvious in this way, inevitability of loss is inaccurately seen as

Activity 10 / 3

10

reducing or removing the pain of bereavement. Additionally, feeling sad is a natural and acknowledged part of the process of grieving.

- One factor valuable to highlight in the list of what helps when listening to bereavement reminiscences is the willingness to respond sensitively to 'repetition of recall': repetition in bereavement reminiscence around the circumstances of death or other type of loss; recalling memories directly related to past life with the deceased, or about a previous home, is one of the main ways bereaved individuals recover from a major loss. In addition, such repetition of recall when focusing on positive memories of the past can offer a restorative value to older people, helping them cope with the here and now.

- Point out that another factor that helps when working with bereavement reminiscence is an understanding and acknowledgement of any cultural influences that play a role in how individuals cope with loss. For example, in some cultures it is believed that a 'good death' is only achieved if set rituals to do with dying and grieving are respected. Relatives of the deceased who do not feel that their loved one experienced a good death may find it harder to come to terms with their loss.

To sum up

The experience of loss for older people encompasses both the death of significant loved ones and the loss of *something* precious in their lives.

Older people can be supported in the grieving process by sensitive responses to the expression of bereavement reminiscence connected to death or other significant loss.

Activity 11 / 1

11

Taking Care of the Carers

MATERIALS NEEDED: Ask group members to bring to the session a photograph or illustration of their favourite place, which does not have to be somewhere they have visited. Flipchart paper for groups of four to six people.

Purpose

1 To emphasize that carers are the greatest resource in all reminiscence work.

2 To look at strategies to overcome personal and organisational blocks to setting up reminiscence programmes.

3 To increase individuals' personal stress recognition.

4 To help individuals identify effective ways to reduce feelings of stress.

What to do

- Explain to the group the purpose of the activity, as outlined above.
- Point out that the reminiscence process cannot be effective, enjoyable and ongoing for older people without the commitment of carers and their managers. Emphasize that, as carers working with older people, individuals are currently coping with rewarding but, at times, physically and emotionally draining work. Feelings of stress are to be expected, and are common when faced with this kind of work.
- The value of reminiscence work to carers and older people is increasingly appreciated, but in order to positively promote the activity, a commitment of time and energy is required. Carers in their role as reminiscence leaders are the most valuable tools within the reminiscence process. To develop and run what may be a new activity within a care setting, ongoing resources and support are essential.
- This part of the group activity is designed to look at how to overcome personal and organisational blocks to setting up a reminiscence programme within care settings. One major block in starting or extending an activity such as

Activity 11 / 2

11

reminiscence work is personal stress felt by carers as a result of their present workload, which reduces time and energy for new commitments. The following are exercises aimed at highlighting how to identify personal stress within the work situation, and how to alleviate its effects.

- Ask group members to write down a personal block and an organisational block that may prevent an effective reminiscence programme being set up within their unit. Group members can do this anonymously, to encourage openness.
- Collect the suggestions and list the blocks highlighted by the group members in two columns, headed 'Personal Blocks' and 'Organisational Blocks'. When the two lists have been drawn up, encourage discussion about the points in each column, highlighting when more than one group member has chosen the same block.
- Lack of time, provoking feelings of stress, may be highlighted as a common personal and organisational block to starting a programme. The work does involve a heavy time commitment, and supervisors need to allow sufficient time for the planning, setting up and running of both one-to-one and group reminiscence.
- Point out that the absence of sufficient time to complete necessary tasks results in a backlog of tasks waiting; the feeling of being undervalued and underpaid for demanding work; the relentlessness and complexity of work that involves the daily lives of others; being at odds with the priorities of management or the wider organisation; feeling that resources are inadequate generally to meet the task. All of these create stress in workers in caring professions.
- With the group, look at a definition of stress: *stress is a physical and/or emotional response to any pressure put upon individuals; it is the way the body tries to restore a normal balance.* Stress is usually associated with being exposed to one or more difficult, overwhelming and worrying experiences. Point out also that exciting or fulfilling experiences can provoke pressure and require adaptation too. In addition, everyone needs some degree of stress in their lives to go on functioning and developing. Problems arise, however, when there is too much stress, resulting from factors such as the constancy of pressure, feeling powerless to change negative situations, and being unsupported in work and personal situations.
- Emphasize that often individuals feel inadequate, due to the complexity of the

Activity 11 / 3 11

task or tasks required of them within the time, skills and resources available. In these instances, personal stress is experienced as a result of unrealistic demands placed on workers by organisations. Being able to recognise when demands are too great, due to organisational practices, helps to alleviate feelings of self-blame, which are a common feature of stress.

- Point out that whatever the initial cause of stress, when it manifests itself at a personal level, its effects have to be handled by individuals. This part of the activity is aimed at identifying how individuals experience stress, and devising strategies for handling its effects.
- Split the large group into small groups of four to six. Ask each group to draw a large stick person on flipchart paper, and indicate on the drawing where and in what form group members' experience the effects of stress. For example, one individual may experience regular headaches at the end of the day and these could be illustrated appropriately on the stick person. If individuals are able to identify the sort of situations that provoke a particular reaction to stress, ask them to write these down as well.
- When completed, display the stick people. As a large group discuss commonalities of stress reactions highlighted, and look together at what provokes stressful feelings.
- In the large group, ask individuals to brainstorm strategies currently used to cope with personal stress, and discuss their effectiveness. The following are some ideas that may be useful to add to the group members' strategies:
  - Acknowledging when the task required is beyond the limits of personal and organisational resources: that is, the level of training, previous experience, general expectations of role, and time available.
  - Asking colleagues for support when tasks are overwhelming.
  - Being assertive as a group with supervisors when, generally, a number of carers find certain tasks beyond their present level of expertise, or difficult to achieve in the time allocated.
  - Trying to work collectively to improve job satisfaction for yourself and others.
  - Not being hard on yourself: dwell on positives and achievements rather than difficulties.

Activity 11 / 4

11

- Recognising when personal stress is building up.
- Avoiding missing set break times, and if feeling stressed a few minutes, where possible, right away from difficult situations can ease tension.
- Building a repertoire of personal de-stressors. For example, a quick break may help during work, while a long chat with a friend may be a strategy for winding down at the end of the day.
- Building into every day at least one personal treat; if life is visualised as a pair of scales, when energy and commitment is taken out on one side of the scales, the other side needs replenishing through rest, treats, relaxing times, positive feedback, and time away from demands, in order to prevent an imbalance in physical and emotional reserves.
- Identifying a personally supportive phrase or image that could be summoned up during stressful periods. If a phrase is chosen, relate it to personal strengths. For example, 'I am able to cope with so many situations, I will find a way to work this out!'; 'I have a lot to offer this work; one mistake does not make me a failure!'
- A chosen image could be of a favourite place that holds pleasurable memories, or somewhere an individual would like to visit. Discuss in the large group why individuals chose their particular favourite places: are there common themes that make the choice appealing, such as a place of beauty, relaxation and escape? Suggest that individuals conjure up this image the next time they feel stressed, to counteract tension.

To sum up

The energy and commitment of carers and their managers to reminiscence work is crucial if it is to play an effective role in the care of older people. Identifying personal and organisational blocks to the introduction of a reminiscence programme is the first step in overcoming difficulties.

Personal stress caused by lack of time, expertise, training and unrealistic organisational demands can be both debilitating and a disincentive to the introduction of innovative work. Acknowledging when and why stress happens, together with developing a toolbox of personal de-stressors, helps to alleviate negative physical and emotional effects of stress.

Evaluation of Activities Form

The training activities have been designed with the aim of building confidence and skills to enable participants to initiate and maintain individual and groupwork reminiscence projects. Please use this evaluation to consider how useful the training has been in your work.

What were your hopes on starting the training? ______________________________

____

____

What are your feelings at the end of the training? ______________________________

____

____

Duration of activities

☐ Too long ☐ About right

Please comment on the balance of practical exercises, discussion and theory input.

☐ Not balanced ☐ Too much emphasis on ______________________________

____

☐ About right

Content of activities

Valuable in increasing general awareness of good practice issues in the care of older people?

☐ Not at all ☐ Partly ☐ Very Valuable

Increased knowledge, confidence and skills in how to initiate reminiscence work with older people?

☐ Not at all ☐ Partially ☐ Greatly

Which activity did you find most useful and why? ______________________________

____

____

____

Evaluation of Activities *continued*

Which activity did you find least useful and why? ____________________

____

____

____

How will you take this training forward into your work? ____________________

____

____

Please tick one or more, or add your own comments:

☐ I am planning to co-run a reminiscence group.

☐ I am planning to do one-to-one reminiscence work.

☐ It will generally improve my awareness, knowledge and skills across all areas of social and emotional care of older people.

Any comments you wish to make about any aspects of the training?

____

____

____

____

____

____

____

____

____

____

____

Name ____________________ Date ____________________

Bibliography

Aristotle, 1995, *Treatise on Rhetoric*, translated by Buckley T, Great Books in Philosophy, Prometheus Books, New York.

Baker F, 1992, *All the Days Ahead: A Testament of Bereavement*, Darton, Longman & Todd, London.

Bennet J, 2000, 'Senior Service', *Independent on Sunday*, 3 December.

Butler R, 1963, 'The life review: interpretation of reminiscence in the aged', *Psychiatry: Journal for the Study of Interpersonal Processes*, Vol 26 (1), pp65–76.

Coleman PG, 1986, 'Ageing and Reminiscence Process: Social and Clinical Implications', John Wiley, Chichester, in Bornat J (ed), 1995, *Reminiscence Reviewed perspectives, evaluations, achievements*, 2nd edn, Open University Press, Buckingham, p16.

Coleman PG, 1991, 'Ageing and life history: the meaning of reminiscence in later life', in Bornat J (ed), 1995, *Reminiscence Reviewed perspectives, evaluations, achievements*, 2nd edn, Open University Press, Buckingham, p79.

Davis R, 1993, *My Journey into Alzheimer's Disease*, Scripture Press, Amersham-on-the-Hill.

Dobrof R, 1984, 'Introduction: A time for reclaiming the past', in Kaminsky M (ed), *The Uses of Reminiscence: New ways of working with older adults*, Haworth Press, New York.

Doka KJ, 1989, 'Disenfranchised Grief: recognising hidden sorrow', in Moss S & Moss M, 'The impact of family deaths on older people', *Bereavement Care*, Winter 1996, Vol 15(3).

Feinstein E, 1994, 'Getting Older', *Selected Poems*, Cacanet Press, Manchester.

Fielden MA, 1990, 'Reminiscence as a therapeutic intervention with sheltered housing residents: A comparative study', *British Journal of Social Work*, Vol 20(1), pp21–44.

Forsyth DR, 1990, *Group Dynamics*, 2nd edn, Brookes/Cole, Pacific Grove, CA.

Friel McGowin D, 1993, *Living in the Labyrinth: A personal journey through the maze of Alzheimer's*, Elder Books, USA.

Gibson F, 1989, *Using Reminiscence: A Training Pack*, Help the Aged, London.

Gibson F, 1998, *Reminiscence and Recall*, 2nd edn, Age Concern, London.

Goldsmith M, Innes A & Kindred M, 1997, in Chapman A (ed), *Hearing the Voice of People with Dementia: A Study Guide*, Dementia Services Development Centre, University of Stirling, Stirling.

Gray Soltys F & Grudzen M, 2000, 'Reminiscence at End of Life: Celebrating a Living Legacy', Dimensions Fall 2000. In an article published on the internet by American Society on Aging http://www.asaging.org.

Hamilton S, in an article in *Reminiscence Magazine*, Age Exchange Theatre Trust, London.

Harris J & Hopkins T, 1995, 'Beyond anti-ageism: Reminiscence groups and the development of anti-discriminatory social work education and practice', in Bornat J (ed), *Reminiscence Reviewed, perspectives, evaluations, achievements*, 2nd edn, Open University Press, Buckingham.

Help the Aged Education Department, 1981, *Recall*, Help the Aged, London.

Kemp M, 1978, *Audio-visual Reminiscence Aids for Elderly People Including the Mentally Frail*, DHSS, London.

Killick J, 1994, *Please Give Me Back My Personality! Writing and Dementia*, Dementia Services Development Centre, University of Stirling, Stirling.

Kitwood T & Bredin K, 1992, *Person to Person*, 2nd edn, Gale Centre Publications, Essex.

Kitwood T & Bredin K, 1997, *The Person Comes First*, Open University Press, Buckingham.

Kunz JA, 1999, *Giving Voice to Lives: Older Adults Publish Life Stories*, in an article published on the internet by National Council of the Aging, Washington DC http://ncoa.org/publications/innovations/Reminiscence%20article.html.

Lendrum S & Syme G, 1994, *Gift of Tears, A Practical Approach to Loss and Bereavement Counselling*, 3rd edn, Routledge, London and New York.

Leick N & Davidsen-Nielsen M, 1991, *Healing Pain: Attachment, Loss and Grief Therapy*, Routledge, London.

Levy A, 2000, 'This is my England', *Guardian*, 19 February.

Lewis CS, 1966, *A Grief Observed*, Faber & Faber, London.

MacArthur D, 1954, 'Nobody Grows Old', *Time*, Vol 63, 24 February.

Mehrabian A, 1972, *Nonverbal Communication*, Aldine-Atherton, Chicago.

Metropolitan Life Insurance Company, 1977, 'Current Patterns of Dependency', *Statistical Bulletin* 58.

Moss SZ & Moss MS, 'The impact of family deaths on older people', *Bereavement Care*, Winter 1996, Vol 15 No 3.

National Heath Strategy, 1991, 'Hospital Services in Australia: access and financing', Melbourne: Commonwealth Department of Health, issues paper no 2 in Hall KA & Hassett AM, 1998, *Assessing and managing old age psychiatric disorders in community practice*, in an article published on the internet by the *Medical Journal of Australia*, http://www.mja.com.au

Randall R & Southgate J, 1980, *Co-operative and Community Group Dynamics... or your meetings needn't be so appalling*, Barefoot Books, London.

Rovner B, Lucas-Blanstein J, Folstein MF & Smith SW, 1990, 'Stability over one year in patients admitted to a nursing home dementia unit', *International Journal of Geriatric Psychiatry*, Vol 5, pp77–82.

Schweitzer P (ed), 1997, *A Place To Stay, Memories of Pensioners from Many Lands*, compiled and published by Age Exchange Theatre Co, London.

Schweitzer P, 1998, '"Routes": A Reminiscence Theatre Project based on the Memories of Older People from the Indian Sub-Continent now Living in Britain', *Reminiscence Magazine*, Spring 1998, Age Exchange Theatre Co, London.

Scrutton S, 1995, *Bereavement and Grief*, Edward Arnold, London, and Age Concern, England.

Thomas B, 2000, *Oral History Conferences*, Oral History Society, in an article published on the internet http://www.nmgw.ac.uk/~ohs/ohs/ohsconfer.html.

Tobin SS, 1991, *Personhood in Advanced Old Age*, Springer, New York.

Wilson E, 2000, 'Building a reminiscence room', *Nursing and Residential Care*, Vol 2, No 11.

Worden JW, 1988, *Grief Counselling and Grief Therapy*, Routledge, London.

Useful Organisations

Agencies offering short training courses in reminiscence work and other courses related to the care of older people

Age Concern Training
Martindale
Hawks Green Lane
Cannock
Staffs WS11 1BR
Tel: 01543 503660
Fax: 01543 504640

Age Exchange Reminiscence Centre/European Reminiscence Network*
11 Blackheath Village
Blackheath
London SE3 9LA
Tel: 020 8318 9105
Fax: 020 8318 0060
Website: www.age-exchange.org.uk
Email: age-exchange@lewisham.gov.uk

Kensington and Chelsea Community History Group*
Methodist Church Centre
240B Lancaster Road
London W11 4AH
Tel: 020 7792 2282
Fax: 020 7792 4426

*Age Exchange, and Kensington and Chelsea Community History Group also run reminiscence group and one-to-one sessions with older people.

Agencies involved in developing oral history work with older people

Oral History Association of America
Baylor University
PO Box 97234
Waco
Texas 76798-7234
Tel: (254) 710 2764
Fax: (254) 710 1571
Website: www.baylor.edu/OHA/Welcome.html

Oral History Society
c/o Department of Sociology
University of Essex
Colchester
Essex CO4 3SQ
Tel: 020 7412 7405
Fax: 020 7412 7441

Victoria Folklife Association
PO Box 1765
Collingwood
Victoria
Australia
Fax: +61 3 9417 4684

Organisations that run national and international conferences on reminiscence

Age Exchange Reminiscence Centre/European Reminiscence Network
see details above

International Institute for Reminiscence and Life Review

University of Wisconsin-Superior	Tel: (715) 394 8469
PO Box 2000	Fax: (715) 394 8381
Superior	Website: http://reminiscenceandlifereview.org
WI 54880-5400	

Oral History Society UK see details above

Oral History Association of America see details above

Organisations offering information on aids and services

Royal National Institute for the Blind

224 Great Portland Street	Tel: 020 7388 1266
London W1N 6AA	

Royal National Institute for Deaf People

105 Gower Street	Tel: 020 7387 8033
London WC1E 6AH	

American Foundation for the Blind

11 Penn Place	Tel: (212) 502 7600
New York	Fax: (212) 502 7777
NY 10001	

Australian Association of the Deaf

Suite 513	Tel: 02 9286 3944
149 Castlereagh Street	Fax: 02 9286 3955
Sydney	
New South Wales 2000	

Alzheimer's Disease Society

Gordon House	Tel: 020 7306 0606
10 Greencoat Place	ADS also runs local carers' support groups.
London SW1P 1PH	

Age Concern England

1268 London Road	Tel: 020 8679 8000
London SW16 4ER	

Counselling agencies

Cruse Bereavement Care
Cruse House
126 Sheen Road
Richmond
Surrey TW9 1UR
Tel: 020 8940 4818
Cruse trains volunteers to work in the community with bereaved individuals.

British Association for Counselling and Psychotherapy
1 Regent Place
Rugby
CV21 2PJ
Tel: 01788 550899
BAC maintains a directory of accredited private counsellors.

Jewish Care
221 Golders Green Road
London NW11 9DW
Tel: 020 8458 3282
Regional information available about counselling for older Jewish people.

Foundation for Black Bereaved Families
11 Kingston Square
Salters Hill
London SE19 1JE
Tel: 020 8661 7228
Offers bereavement counselling and support.

Specialist publications

Journal of Dementia Care
Hawker Publications
13 Park House
140 Battersea Road
London SW11 4NB
Tel: 020 7720 2108
Fax: 020 7498 3023

Reminiscence Magazine
Age Exchange/European Reminiscence Network see details above

Dimensions
American Society of Aging
833 Market Street
San Francisco
CA 94103
Website: www.asaging.org

ONE OF A KIND: The Caregiver's Voice Magazine
Contact: Thelma Kramer
PO Box 3884
Seal Beach
CA 90740-7884

Dementia Services Development Centre
University of Stirling
Stirling
Scotland FK9 4LA
Tel: 01786 467740
Fax: 01786 466846
Books, training packs, videos and audiotapes on issues connected with dementia and older people.

Index